# Rajatsubhra's Manual Opening of Phimosis [RMOP]

Dr Rajatsubhra Mukhopadhyay
Dch, MD[Child][UCN], PGPN Global[BUSM,Medinscribe]

**Child Health Care Arambag,**
Koruna Medical, Hospital More, Arambag,
Hooghly, West Bengal, India, Pin-712601
e-mail:dr_rajatsubhra@sridoctor.com
Phone : 9732948496
Web site: http://www.sridoctor.com

**Residence: Konarpur. Po-Sihar, Dist-Bankura.Pin-722161. WB. India.**

### BOOK 'S INFORMATION DETAILS:

- **Paperback:** 74 pages
- **Publisher:** CreateSpace Independent Publishing Platform; First Edition,Volume 1 (September 5, 2018)
- **ISBN-13: 978-1727057003**
- **SIZE: 8.5" x 11" on COLOR Paper**

Please follow and inspire the CREATIVITY by advising to follow:
**my other books** by Amazon. https://www.amazon.in/Dr-Rajatsubhra-Mukhopadhyay-MD/e/B007HJ0F70.
My Videos in YOU Tube:
https://www.youtube.com/results?search_query=therajatsubhra
My WEB SITE: http://www.sridoctor.com
My BLOG: https://indologyblog.blogspot.com/
My Professional page in Face book:
 https://www.facebook.com/Child-Health-Care-Arambag-115522941862665/

## TOPIC

| | |
|---|---|
| PREFACE | 4-6 |
| ACKNOWLEDGEMENT | 7 |

## RMOP[Rajatsubhra's Manual Opening of Phimosis]

| | |
|---|---|
| INTRODUCTION | 8 |
| KEY POINTS and OBJECTIVES | 9 |
| SUMMERY | 10 |
| METHOD | 11-15 |
| STATISTICS | |
| DISCUSSION | 16-17 |
| CONCLUSION | 18 |
| REFERRENCE | 19-20 |
| DATA | 38-64 |

Please follow and inspire the CREATIVITY by advising to follow:
**my other books** by Amazon. https://www.amazon.in/Dr-Rajatsubhra-Mukhopadhyay-MD/e/B007HJ0F70:

My Videos in YOU Tube:
https://www.youtube.com/results?search_query=therajatsubhra

My WEB SITE: http://www.sridoctor.com

My BLOG: https://indologyblog.blogspot.com/

My Professional page in Face book:
https://www.facebook.com/Child-Health-Care-Arambag-115522941862665/

# PREFACE

## Rajatsubhra's Manual Opening of Phimosis[RMOP]

I was trying to publish a paper on Manual Opening of Phimosis since 2009. But today's medico legal situation, insufficiency of support to publish original work from a remote rural set up, fear of sabotage and lack of infrastructure all put the mater into a failure.

*Still from the remote rural area I am trying to continue an academic life and this great Publishing platforms are the way left to preserve my claim over the concept of the procedure used [RMOP]Rajatsubhra's Manual Opening of Phimosis , will be beneficial to the society in future.*

This book is a product of all those days and effort. This is indeed a tremendous difficult job to me to do all the works of publishing of this book by myself and it will never be possible without the generous help of the Members of the CREATE SPACE. Starting from the cover design, interior and publishing channel setup everything is guided by their novel system and help. You are not only reader, you are thinker and the judge of my effort. All of yours supports are very important to me.

Phimosis is a natural phenomenon. Usually it opens up .

But those who faces difficulty may pass through prolonged massaging and prepusoplasty or Circumcision is advised. This common advises I have come acrossed several times in my professional life.

 I decided to find out a solution of it so that surgery can be totally avoided.

Steroid has a keratostatic and skin thinning effect and Salysilic Acid has a keratolytic effect [reference is given inside].

 I use it for few days to help my Non Surgical and Manual Procedure . I use it for a short course to avoid any systemic side effect. [This is also readily available for treatment of different skin problem like Atopic Dermatitis, Lichen Planus etc. in child. ]

Now I am completely successful in my own innovative, easy and cost effective method. This is a painless, bloodless tactics. This takes only few seconds to learn and needs a good practice .I have named it RMOP[Rajatsubhra's Manual Opening of Phimosis].

*This book is being published to preserve my claim on this procedure and concept.*

# ACKNOWLEDGEMENT

I am grateful to CREATE SPACE for providing such a beautiful platform to publish this book. I also thanks Google Image for many images collected for this book.

Lastly thanks to my wife and family who always support and encourage me for this critical job done by self after busy medical life from this rural set up.

With regards,
Dr Rajatsubhra Mukhopadhyay
Dch, MD[Child][UCN], PGPN Global[BUSM,Medinscribe].
4.9.2018

Please follow and inspire the CREATIVITY by advising to follow:
**my other books** by Amazon. https://www.amazon.in/Dr-Rajatsubhra-Mukhopadhyay-MD/e/B007HJ0F70.
My Videos in YOU Tube: https://www.youtube.com/results?search_query=therajatsubhra
My WEB SITE: http://www.sridoctor.com
My BLOG: https://indologyblog.blogspot.com/
My Professional page in Face book: https://www.facebook.com/Child-Health-Care-Arambag-115522941862665/

## INTRODUCTION:

PHIMOSIS is non reducibility of penile foreskin or prepuce. This may be Physiological or Pathological.[1]

Physiological: Since birth it is seen in almost every children upto three years. It is normal.[2] [3] After that it is advised to open this with massaging, Prepuceplasty or Circumcision. But this could be opened with different technique without surgery.

Pathological: This could also be used in pin hole meatus and after scarring from Balanitis.[3]

Opening is important because of regular washing of the Smegma. As this is supposed to have carcinogenic property. [4] Otherwise, there is a chance of fungal infection. So daily hygienic care is important. In latter life, for conjugal life this is very important.

A open level double blinded randomized case control study was done with 100 patient receiving this treatment and control was 50 patients who received massaging with steroid ointment.

1. Measured association in Chi Square Test
P value in
Mid P exact with Degree of Freedom[DF] =1 is 0.00002019 [1 tail]
P value in
McNemar test: 0.00004458[2 tail], Value : 16.67

2. Pair matched Odds Ratio: Point Estimate :2. At 95% confidence interval s
lower limit : 1.424, upper limit: 2.808[Taylor series]

Both are statistically very significant.

**KEY WORDS**:
Phimosis, Short Course Topical Steroid- Salicylic Acid Therapy

**OBJECTIVES:**
The aim of study is to find out more easier approach to Phimosis,. This will in terms help to manage Pin hole Meatus, Urethritis, UTI. It will decrease the cost, post operative stage and need of surgery also.

## SUMMERY:

During office practice among all male children above 1 years of age with Phimosis, for past years the author advised his own method [Rajatsubhra's Manual Opening of Phimosis: RMOP] to open the Phimosis. All of them have success. None required surgery. A open level double blinded randomized case control study was done with 100 patient receiving this treatment and control was 50 patients who received massaging with steroid ointment.

1. Measured association in Chi Square Test
 P value in
Mid P exact with Degree of Freedom[DF] =1 is 0.00002019 [1 tail]
P value in
McNemar test: 0.00004458[2 tail], Value : 16.67
2. Pair matched Odds Ratio: Point Estimate :2. At 95% confidence interval s
lower limit : 1.424, upper limit: 2.808[Taylor series]
Both are statistically very significant.
This shows this manual opening method [RMOP]is better option for opening phimosis.

# METHOD

**TYPE OF STUDY** : non randomized active controlled trial
**INTERVENTION NAME**- Rajatsubhra's Manual Opening of Phimosis[RMOP].
CONTROLLED INTERVENTION NAME- Comparison between two groups with manual opening after application of steroid –Salicylic acid ointment & Massaging after application of steroid ointment. Both of the groups having Phimosis.

**INCLUSIONS CRITERIA:** 1. Age above 1year. 2. Pin hole meatus. 3. Balanitis. 4. Ballooning.

**EXCLUSIONS CRITERIA:** 1. Age group below 6 month of age. 2. with out written consent. 3. with other acute illness.

There was no method of generating **randomization sequence** as this was a non randomized trial.
Method of **allocation concealment** is not applicable.

**BLINDING & MASKING** -OPEN LABEL. As there was no stoppage of intervention of masking

Total patients 150. Sets in two groups. Group 1. 100 Patients with steroid and salicylic acid application followed by done RMOP. Group2. 50 patients using steroid ointment for massage for one month. In first group 100 out of 100 was opened up. 2. In second group 15out of 50 was opened up.
Whenever more than 1 year old male patient comes to the clinic the author have a routine check up for Phimosis. And if it is seen then they are advised to apply topical steroid [Mometasone] with salicylic acid only for seven days & for seven times. The steroid has a skin thinning effect.[5,6,7]. Salicylic Acid has also skin thinning effect.[8]. The consent of the parents in written format is kept for every patients. Followed by usage of topical lignocaine 2% half an hour prior to visit the doctor. Then a gentle repeated traction with a little skill makes the fore skin opened. Smegmas comes as white cheesy matter. Usage of Povidone Iodine is done to make it clear. Followed by usage of an antibiotic ointment for another three to four days & regular washing as an hygienic care during bathe makes it normal. After opening of phimosis and success the remarks are collected from every parents.

. With a short course of topical steroid, none is affected from steroid 's side effects. This is named as RMOP[Rajatsubhra's Manual opening of Phimosis.]
The addition of Salicylic acid and manual opening is newer here in this study. Use of Steroid was previously done. [9]

### NOTE:
the author have used a potent topical steroid [Mometasone]; but with mild steroid, other keratolytic agents study have to be done.

### CONSENT:
The consent of the parents in written format is kept for every patients. After opening of phimosis and success the remarks are collected from every parents.

## STATISTICAL DATA ANALYSIS:

In Group 1. [manual opening with steroid-salicylic acid ointment]
    Total Case: ........................100
    Success............................ 100

Easy to open 60
Difficult 40.

On first chance 97
$2^{nd}$ chance 2
$3^{rd}$ chance 1.

...................Complication:...............................................……

Bleeding 30
Cry 99
Swelling 20
Paraphimosis 20
Erosion 50
Infection 0
………………..Rephimosis……………..20

Cases [Patients with steroid –Salicylic acid and manual opening] = 100 Success= 100
Control [Patients with steroid ointments and massaging]= 50. .Success = 15.

## MATCHED PAIR CASE CONTROL TABLE
### Single Table Analysis

|      |   | CONTROL + | CONTROL − | TOTAL |
|------|---|-----------|-----------|-------|
| CASE | + | 100       | 100       | 200   |
|      | − | 50        | 35        | 85    |
|      |   | 150       | 135       | 285   |

### Measures of Association

| Test | Value | d.f. | P Values 1-tail | 2-tail |
|---|---|---|---|---|
| McNemar: | 16.67 | 1 |  | 0.00004458 |
| McNemar with continuity correction: | 16.01 | 1 |  | 0.00006315 |
| Fisher exact |  |  | 0.00002724 | 0.00005448 |
| Mid-P exact |  |  | 0.00002019 | 0.00004037 |

There are 150 discordant pairs.
Because this number is >= 20, the McNemar test can be used.

## Odds-based Estimates

| Parameter | Point Estimate | 95% Confidence Intervals Lower,Upper | Type |
|---|---|---|---|
| Pair-Matched Odds Ratio: | 2 | 1.424, 2.808[1] | Taylor series |
| CMLE Odds Ratio* | 2 | 1.429, 2.826[1] | Mid-P Exact |
|  |  | 1.411, 2.868[1] | Fisher Exact |

*Conditional **maximum likelihood estimate of Odds Ratio**

**(P)indicates a one-tail P-value for Protective or negative association; otherwise one-tailed exact P-values are for a positive association.**

Martin,D; Austin,H (1991) An efficient program for computing conditional maximum likelihood estimates and exact confidence limits for a common odds ratio. Epidemiology 2, 359-362.

Results from OpenEpi, Version 3, open source calculator--MatchCC
Print from the browser with ctrl-P
or select text to copy and paste to other programs.

## DISCUSSION:

From this open level double blinded randomized case control study with 100 patient receiving this treatment and control group with 50 patients who received massaging with steroid ointment this is statistically proved that RMOP is a better rather a method of choice.

1. Measured association in Chi Square Test
 P value in
Mid P exact with Degree of Freedom[DF] =1 is 0.00002019 [1 tail]
P value in
McNemar test: 0.00004458[2 tail],   Value : 16.67

2. Pair matched Odds Ratio: Point Estimate :2. At 95% confidence interval s
lower limit : 1.424,  upper limit: 2.808[Taylor series]

Both are statistically very significant.

TOTAL CASE SENERIO:
In group1 [manual opening with steroid-salicylic acid ointment]
Total Case: ........................100
          Success............................ 100

Easy to open  60
Difficult 40.

On first chance 97
$2^{nd}$ chance 2
$3^{rd}$ chance 1.

..................**Complication**:................................................
......

Early : Bleeding 30

Cry 99
Late:
Swelling 20
Paraphimosis 20

Mild Transient Erosion .50
Infection 0
Rephimosis 20


Paraphimosis : This was seen in 20 patients.
 This is very important complication because of its pain , uneasiness &appearance.  It is occurred for faulty technique to reduce the prepuce/fear to reduce the prepuce. This is tackled with simple assurance & needling to collected fluid spaces & a gentle pressure over it. Followed by gradual retraction done.

Swelling :
 This is also common. For that to use the ointment is advised to apply over the prepuce with out open it..after  subsequent reduction of swelling ,the prepuce is opened & the ointment is applied inside. This could avoid paraphimosis .I found 20 such cases in this study.

Re -Phimosis: from Scarring .  This complication happens occasionally. But could be re opened. This second time it is easier to open. Mild steroid antibiotic ointment is applied to avoid this for seven days two times. There were 20 patients with rephimosis.

## CONCLUSION:

Significance is high. In percentage: 100% success.
The commonest early complication is Bleeding 30%.
The commonest late complication is Mild Transient Erosion. 50%.
This will in terms help to manage all types of Phimosis including Pin hole Meatus, Urethritis and causing UTI. It will decrease the cost, post operative stage and need of surgery also. Sourge RMOP [Rajatsubhra's Manual Opening of Phimosis] is an effective method of treatment for Phimosis.

## REFERRENCES

1. http://urology.ucsf.edu/sites/urology.ucsf.edu/files/uploaded-files/basic-page/phimosis.pdf

2. https://www.ncbi.nlm.nih.gov/pubmed/9316279

3. http://intactwiki.org/wiki/Phimosis

4. http://www.cancer.org/cancer/penilecancer/detailedguide/penile-cancer-risk-factors

5. Lehmann P, Zheng P, Lavker RM, Kligman AM. Corticosteroid atrophy in human skin: a study by light, scanning, and transmission electron microscopy. *J. Invest. Derm.* 1983; 81:169-76.

6. Zheng P, Lavker RM, Lehman P., Kligman AM. Morphologic investigations on the rebound phenomenon after corticosteroid-induced atrophy in human skin. *J. Invest. Derm.* 1984;82: 345-52.

7. Ponec M, De Kloet ER, Kempenaar JA. Corticoids and human fibroblasts: intracellular specific binding in relation to growth inhibition. *J. Invest. Derm.* 1980;75:293-6.

8. https://en.m.wikipedia.org/wiki/Medical_uses_of_salicylic_acid

9. http://www.cirp.org/library/treatment/phimosis/dewan/

RELATED WORKS.

1. https://www.ncbi.nlm.nih.gov/pubmed/16285358

2. https://www.ncbi.nlm.nih.gov/pmc/articles/PMC3329654/

3. https://www.ncbi.nlm.nih.gov/pubmed/10444134
4. https://www.sciencedirect.com/topics/medicine-and-dentistry/phimosis

# CASE DATA

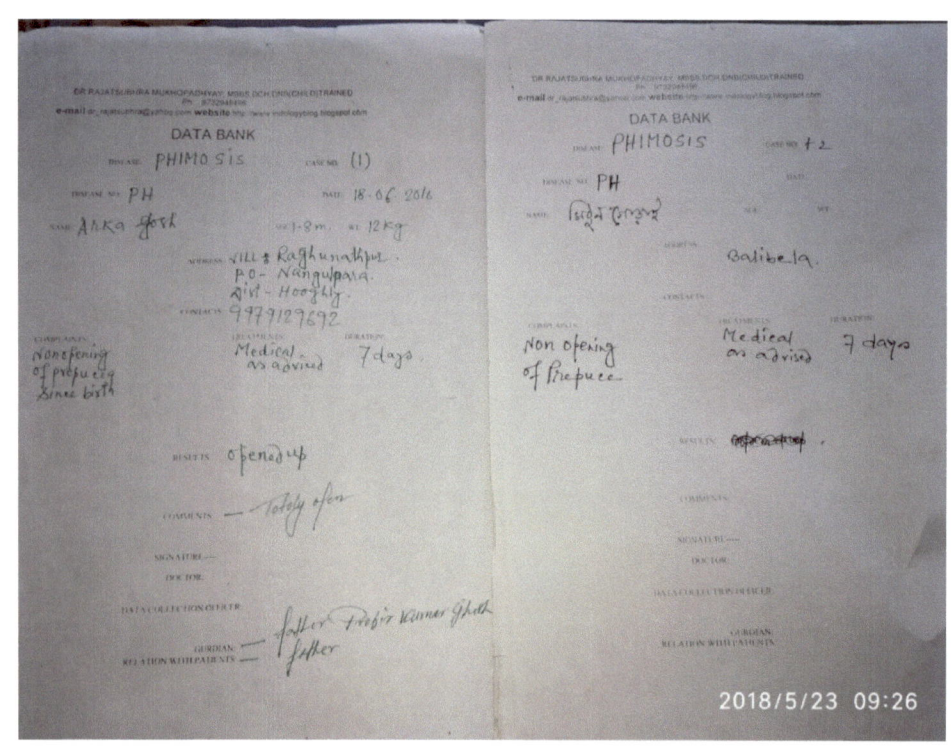

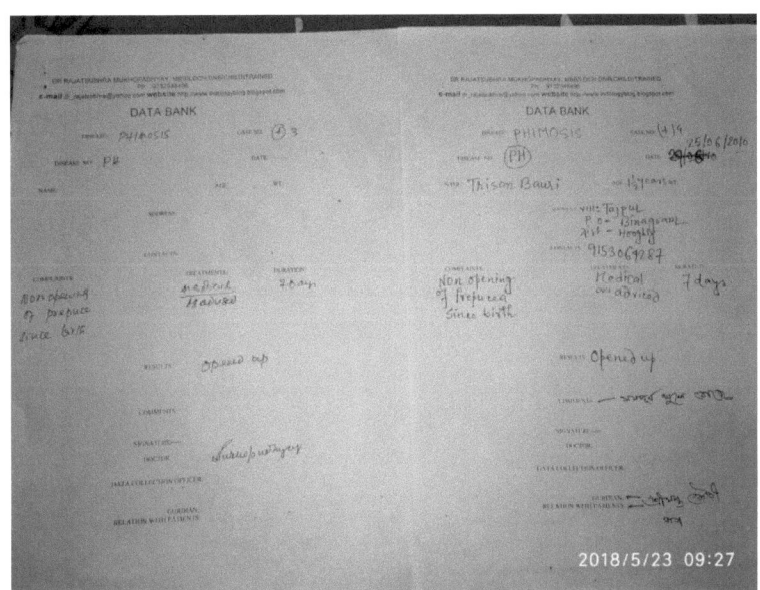
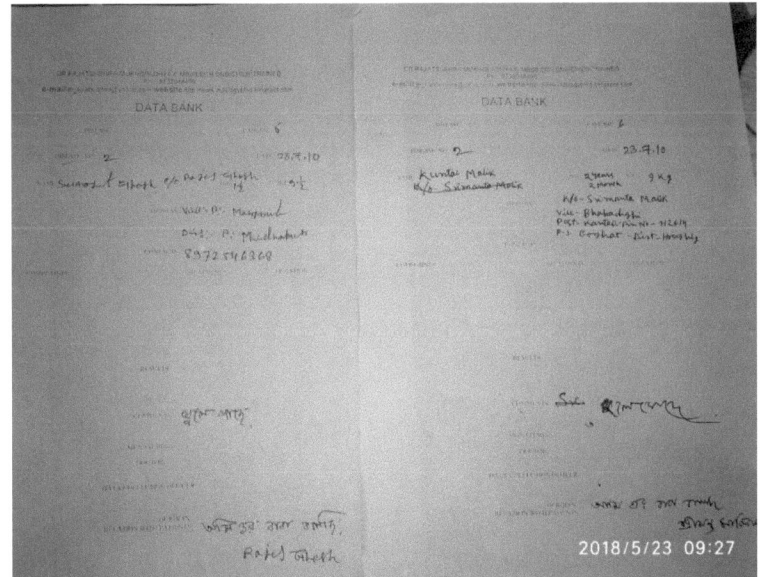

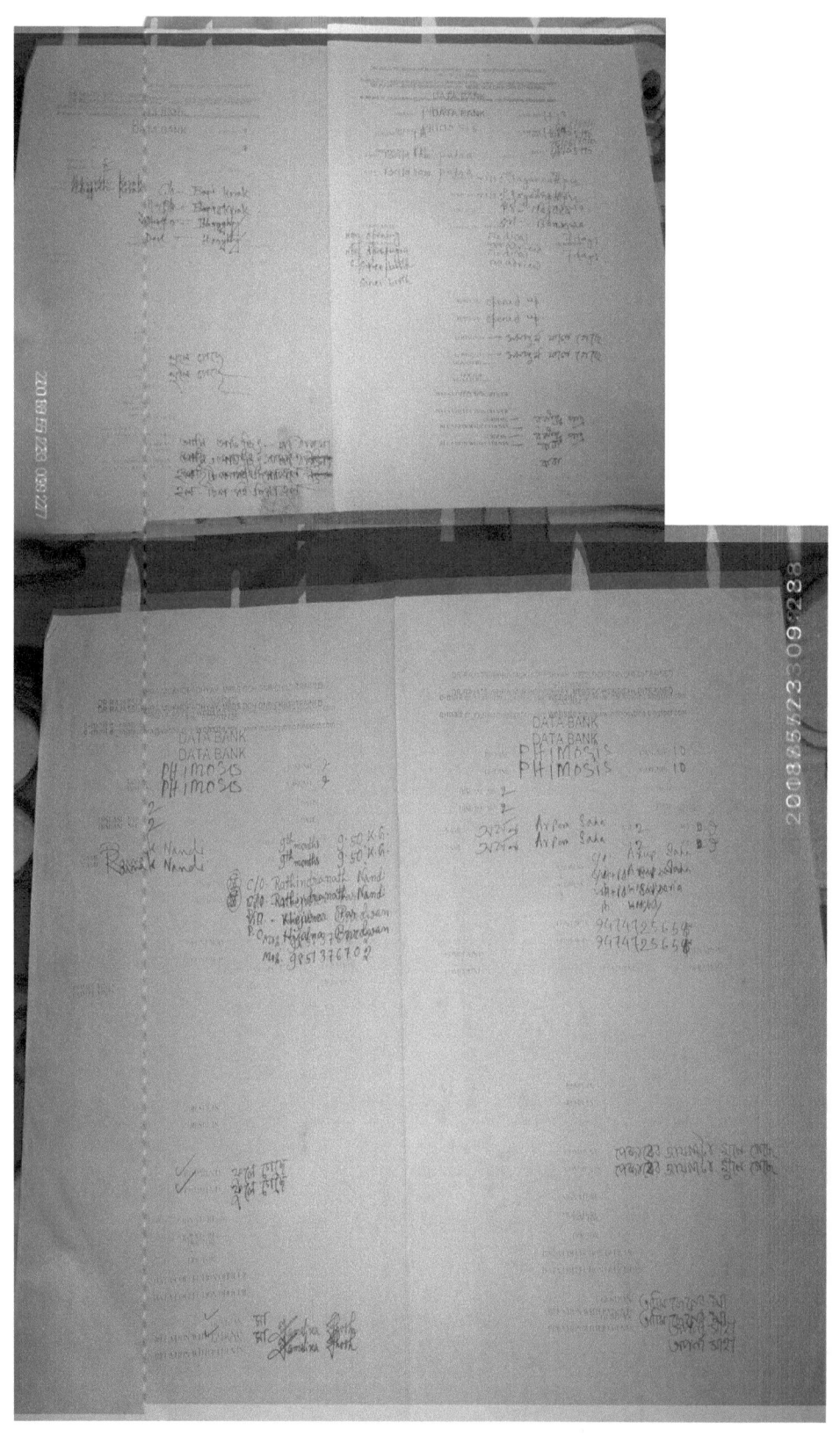

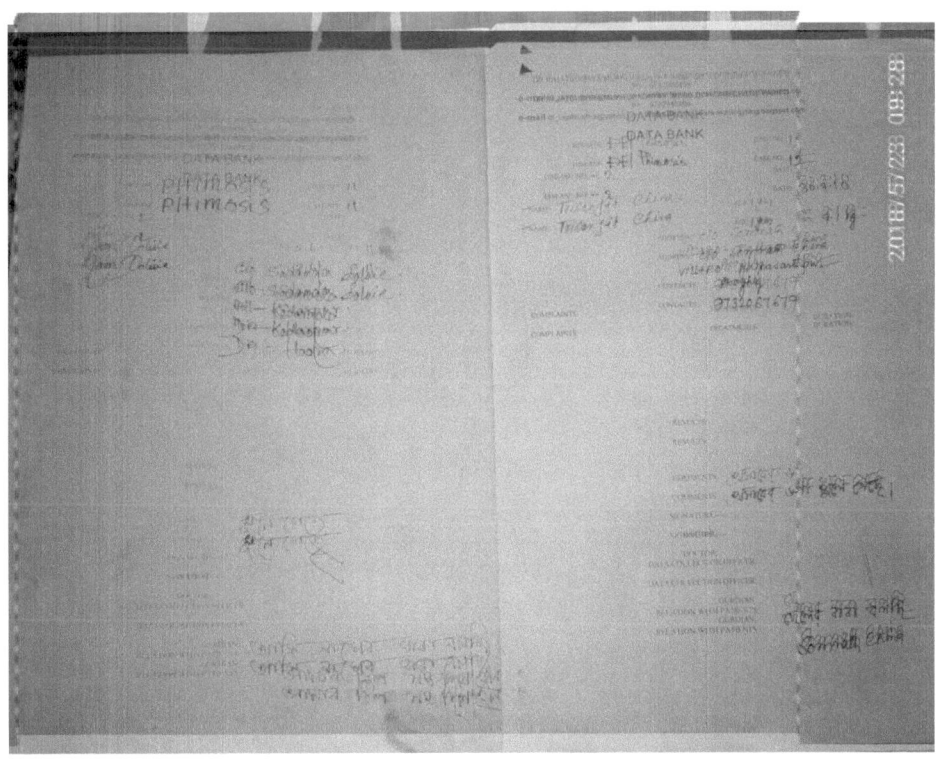

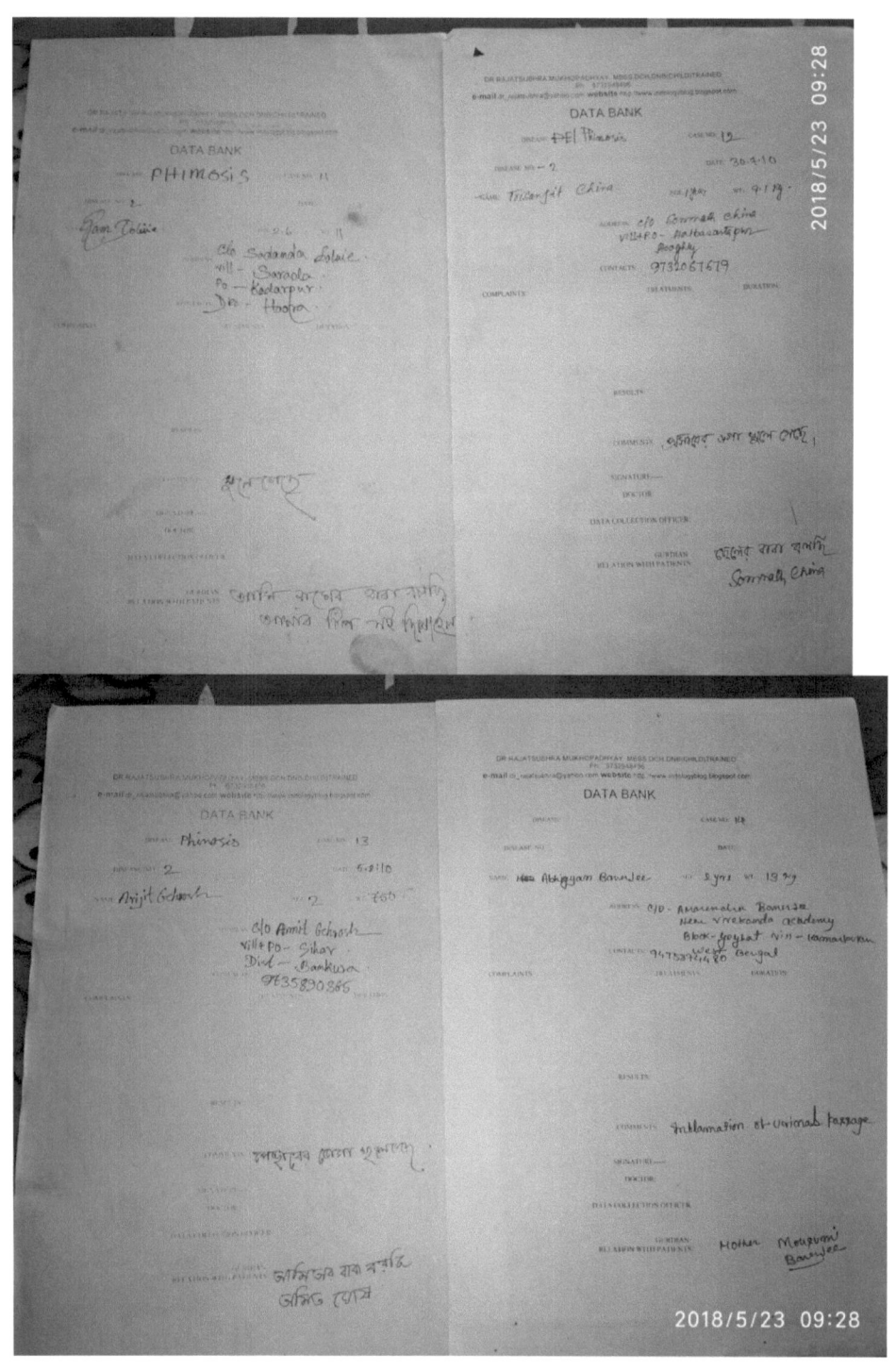

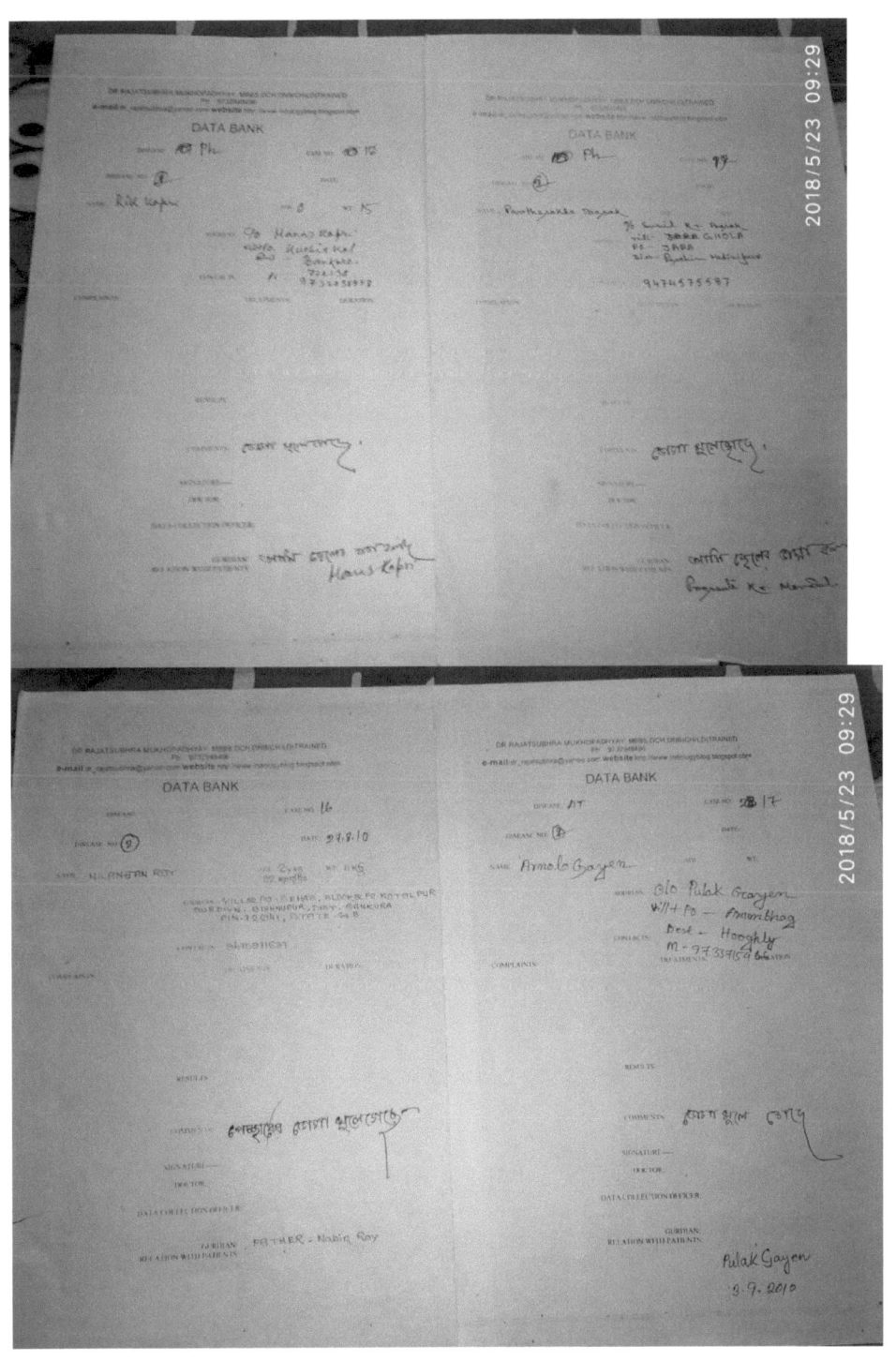

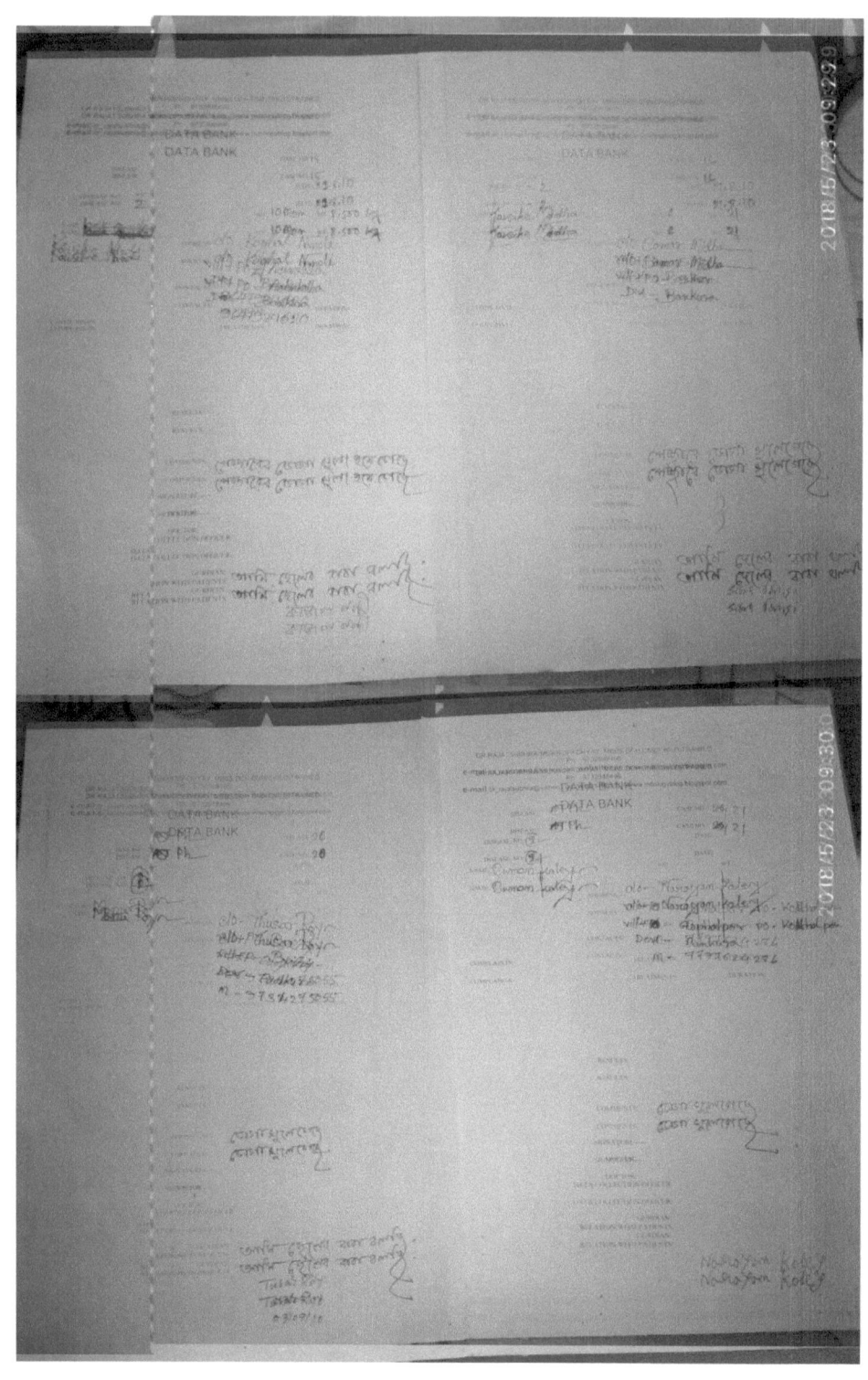

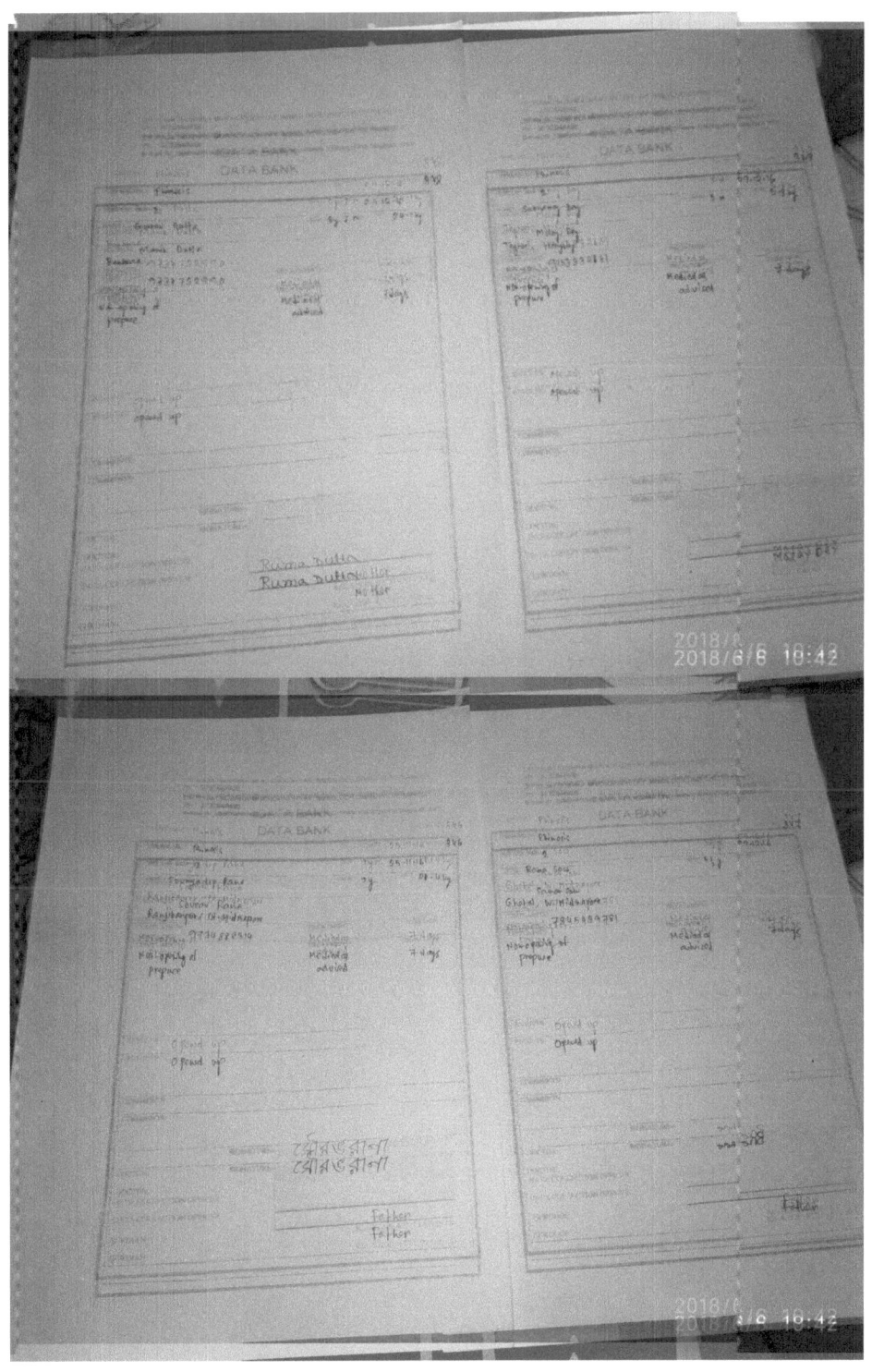

28

29

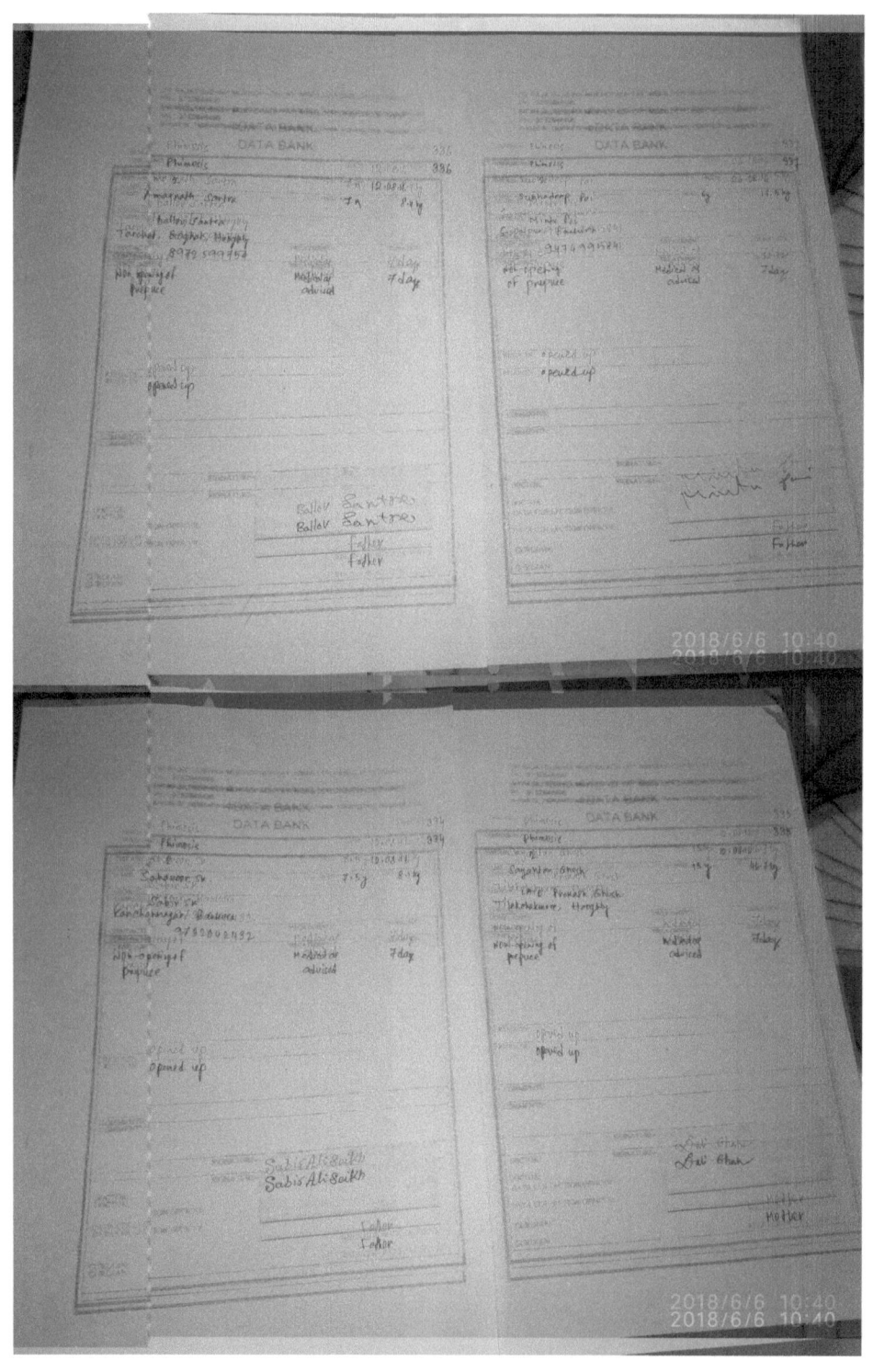

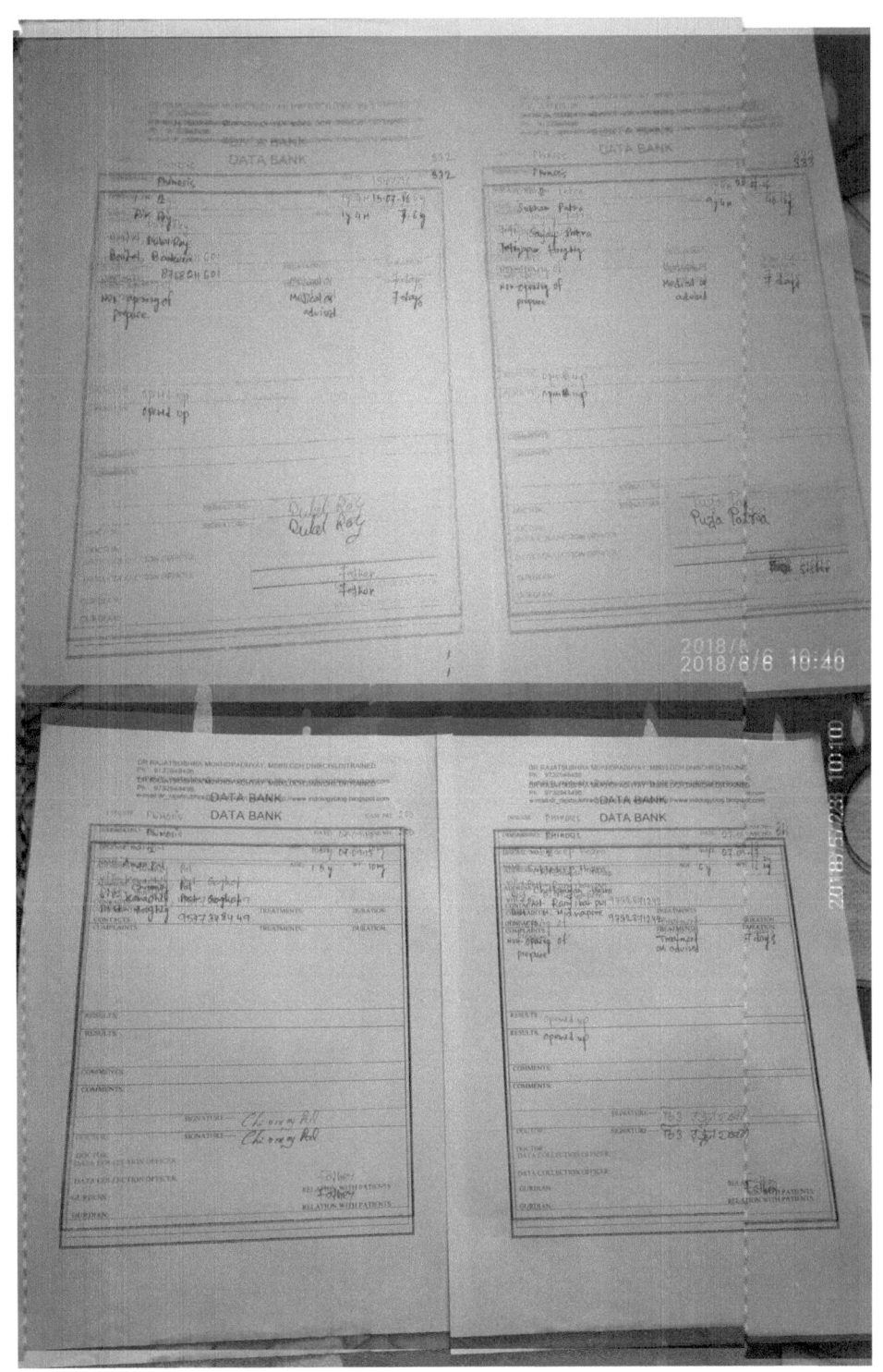

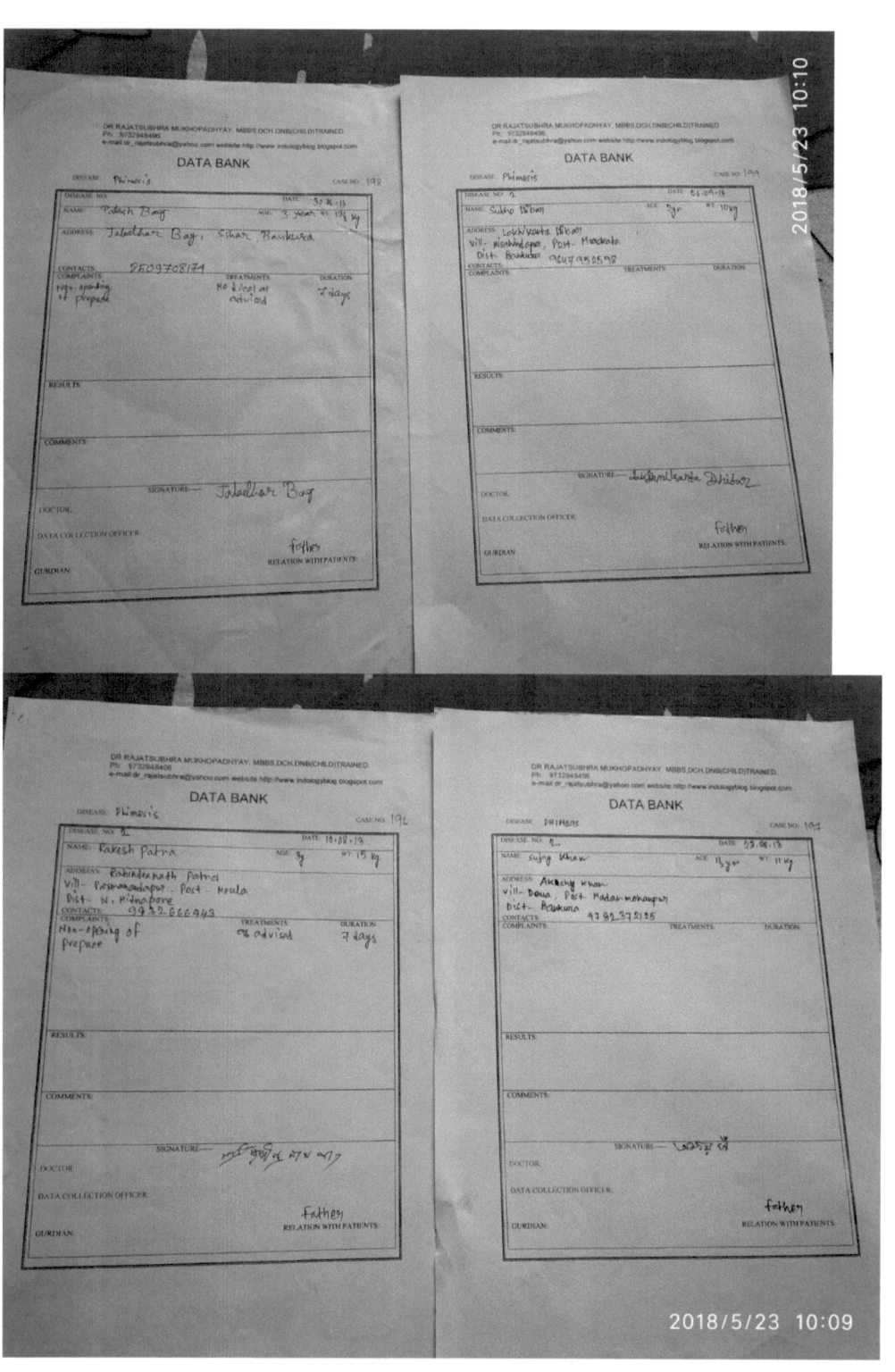

## DATA BANK

**DISEASE:** Phimosis  **CASE NO:** 194
**DISEASE NO.:** 2  **DATE:** 09-08-13
**NAME:** Trishith Roy  **AGE:** 5y  **WT:** 11 kg
**ADDRESS:** Tarun Roy, Vill- Samaspur, Post- Hati, Dist- Hooghly
**CONTACTS:** 9732-612682
**COMPLAINTS / TREATMENTS / DURATION:**

**RESULTS:**
**COMMENTS:**
**SIGNATURE:** Tarun Roy
**DOCTOR:**
**DATA COLLECTION OFFICER:**
**GUARDIAN:** father  **RELATION WITH PATIENTS**

---

## DATA BANK

**DISEASE:** Phimosis  **CASE NO:** 121
**DISEASE NO.:** 2  **DATE:** 09-08-13
**NAME:** Iran Kotal  **AGE:** 1y 9m  **WT:** 10 kg
**ADDRESS:** Raju Kotal, Vill- Balitha, Post- DD, Dist- Bankura
**CONTACTS:** 9659546669
**COMPLAINTS / TREATMENTS / DURATION:**

**RESULTS:**
**COMMENTS:**
**SIGNATURE:**
**DOCTOR:**
**DATA COLLECTION OFFICER:**
**GUARDIAN:**  **RELATION WITH PATIENTS**

---

## DATA BANK

**DISEASE:** Phimosis  **CASE NO:** 192
**DISEASE NO.:** 2  **DATE:** 12-07-13
**NAME:** Arnab Chatterjee  **AGE:** 6m  **WT:** 8 kg
**ADDRESS:** Amiya Chatterjee, Vill- Jikyti, Post- Jayaanti, Dist- Bankura
**CONTACTS:** 9474908751
**COMPLAINTS:** Non-opening of prepuce  **TREATMENTS:** Medical as advised  **DURATION:** 7 days

**RESULTS:**
**COMMENTS:**
**SIGNATURE:** Amiya Chatterjee
**DOCTOR:**
**DATA COLLECTION OFFICER:**
**GUARDIAN:** father  **RELATION WITH PATIENTS**

---

## DATA BANK

**DISEASE:** Phimosis  **CASE NO:** 193
**DISEASE NO.:** 2  **DATE:** 12-07-13
**NAME:** Sourav Choudhury  **AGE:** 1y  **WT:** 9.5 kg
**ADDRESS:** Pintu Choudhury, Vill- Tarhaghati, Post- Paikrajhitha, Dist- W. Midnapore
**CONTACTS:** 88012-72796
**COMPLAINTS:** Non-opening of prepuce  **TREATMENTS:** Medical as advised  **DURATION:** 7 days

**RESULTS:**
**COMMENTS:**
**SIGNATURE:** Pintu Choudhury
**DOCTOR:**
**DATA COLLECTION OFFICER:**
**GUARDIAN:** father  **RELATION WITH PATIENTS**

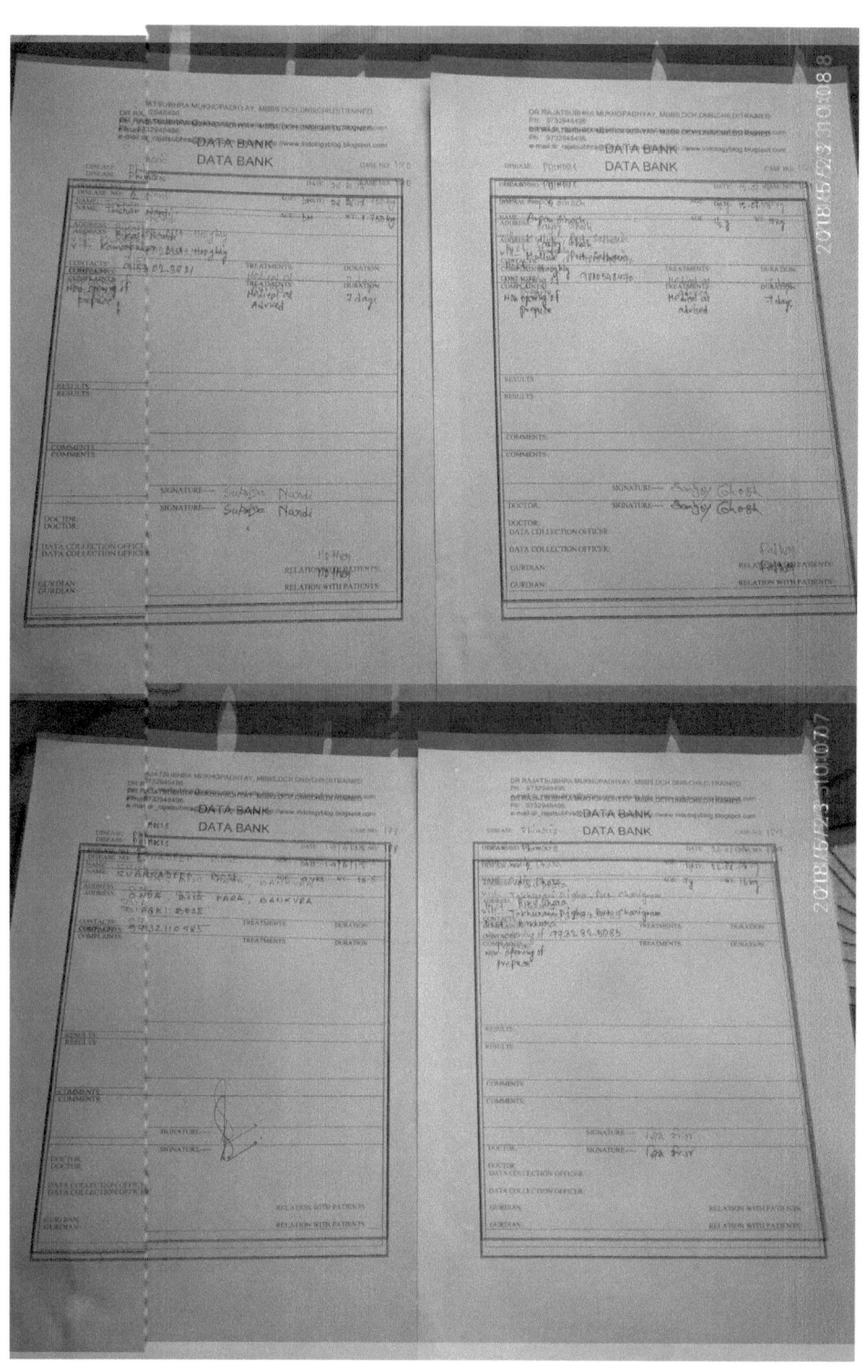

37

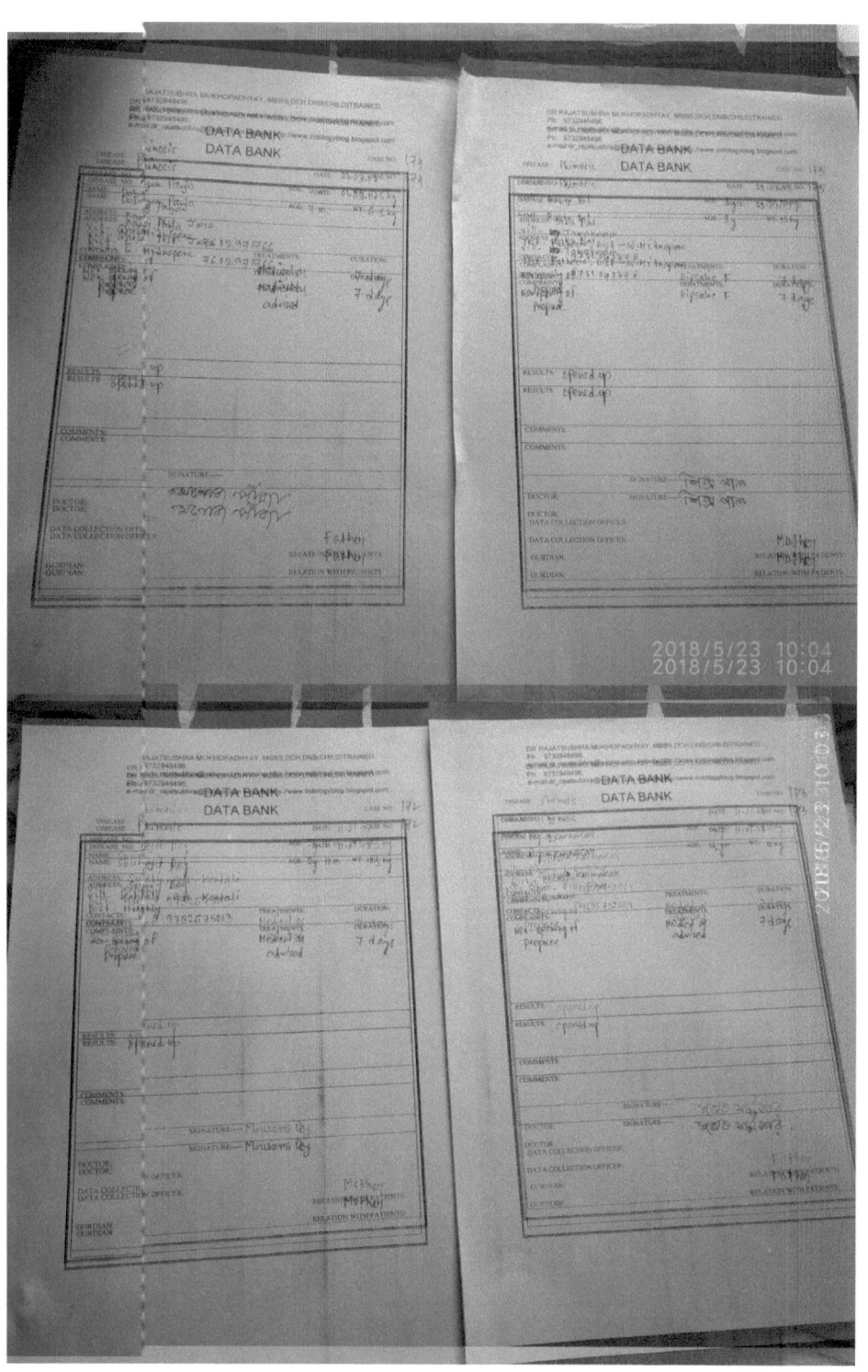

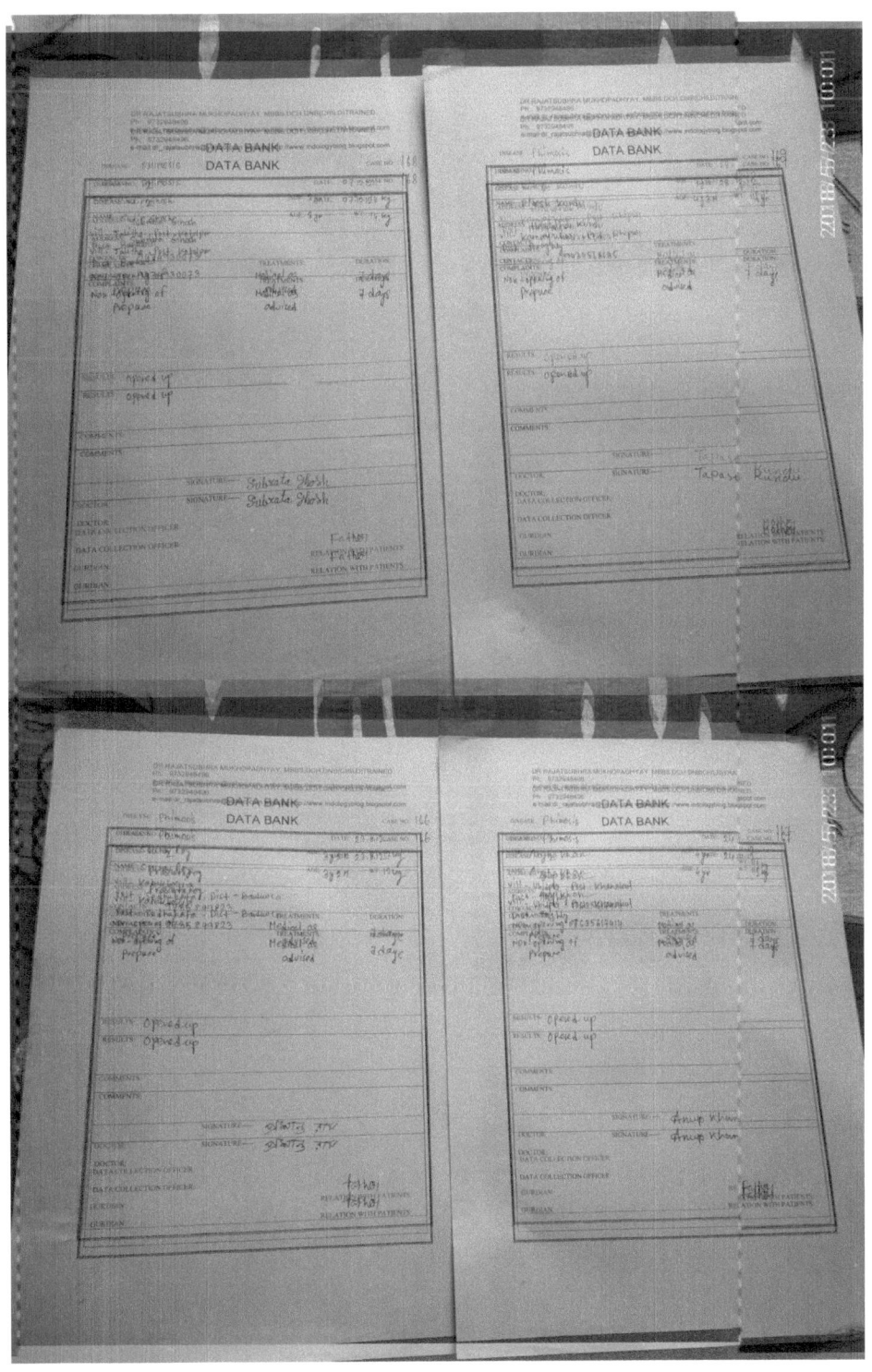

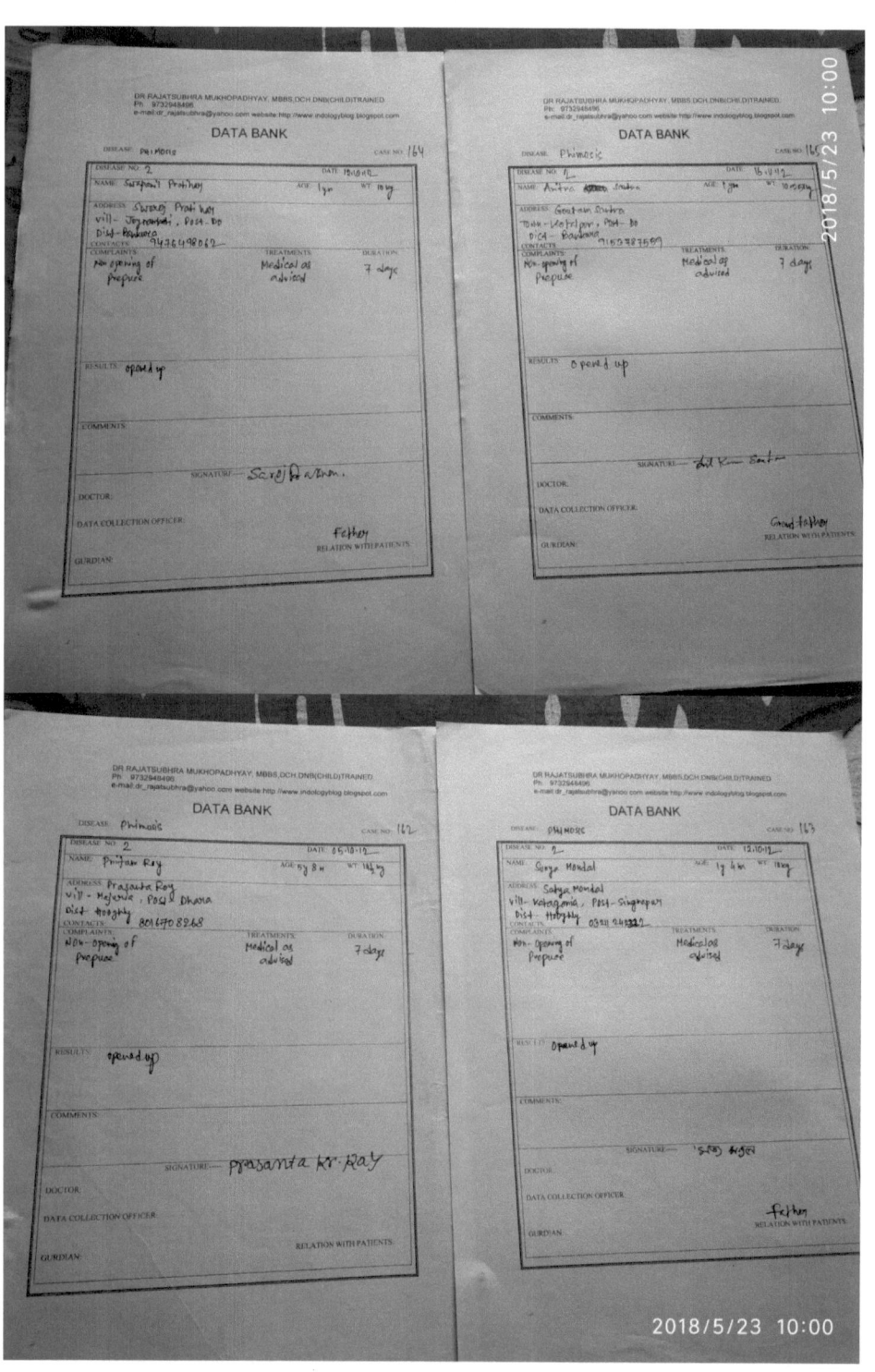

41

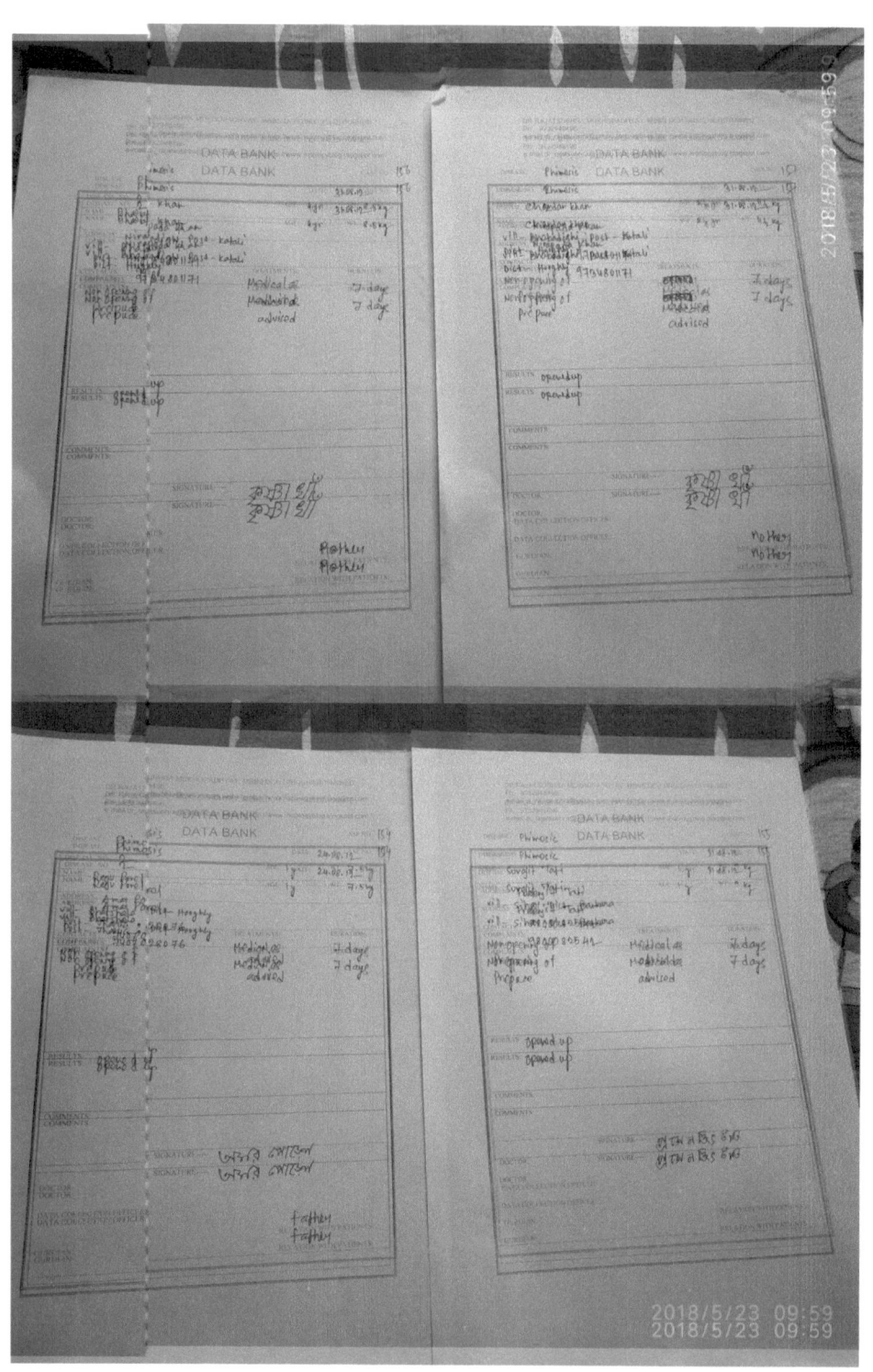

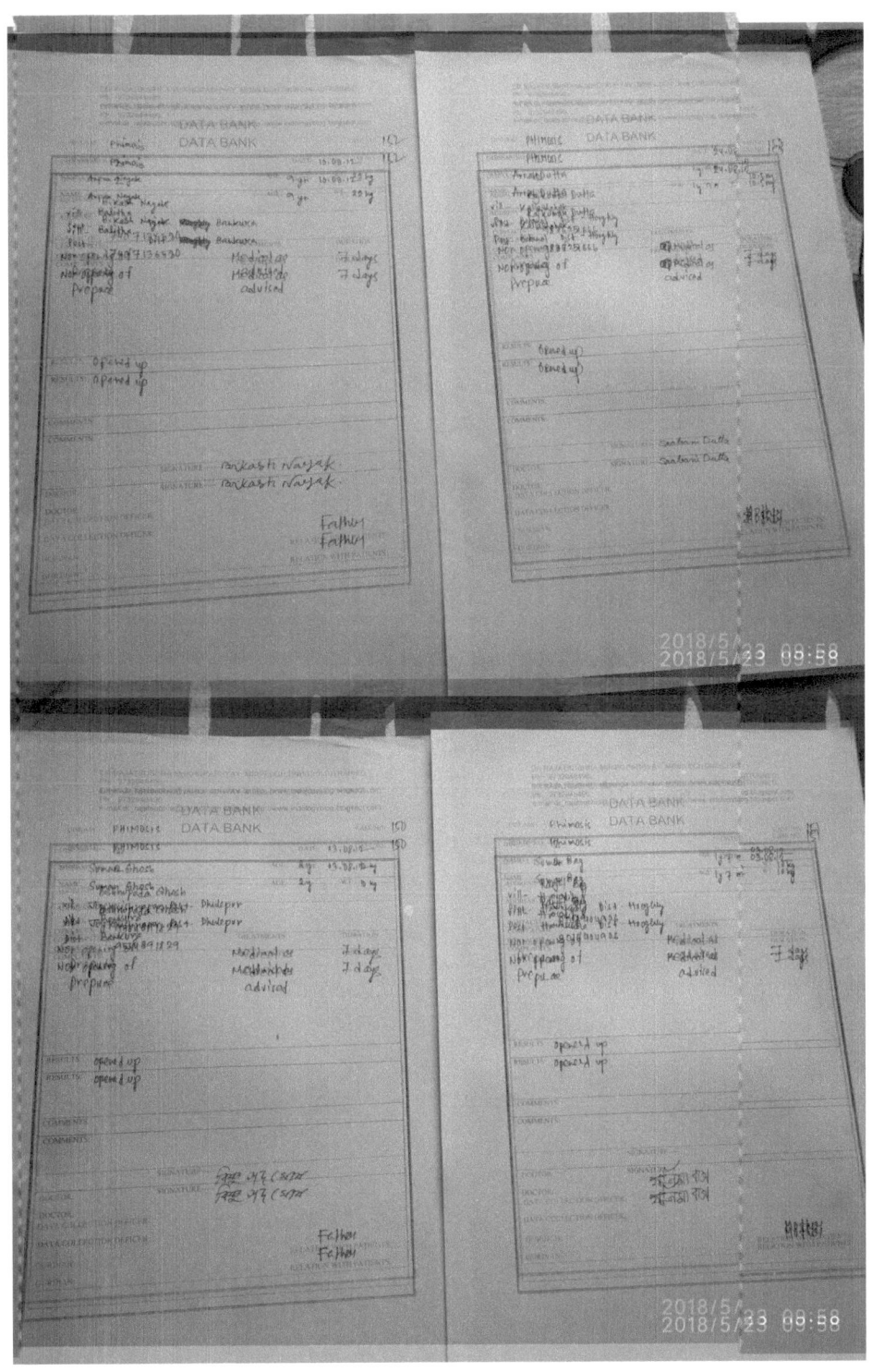

45

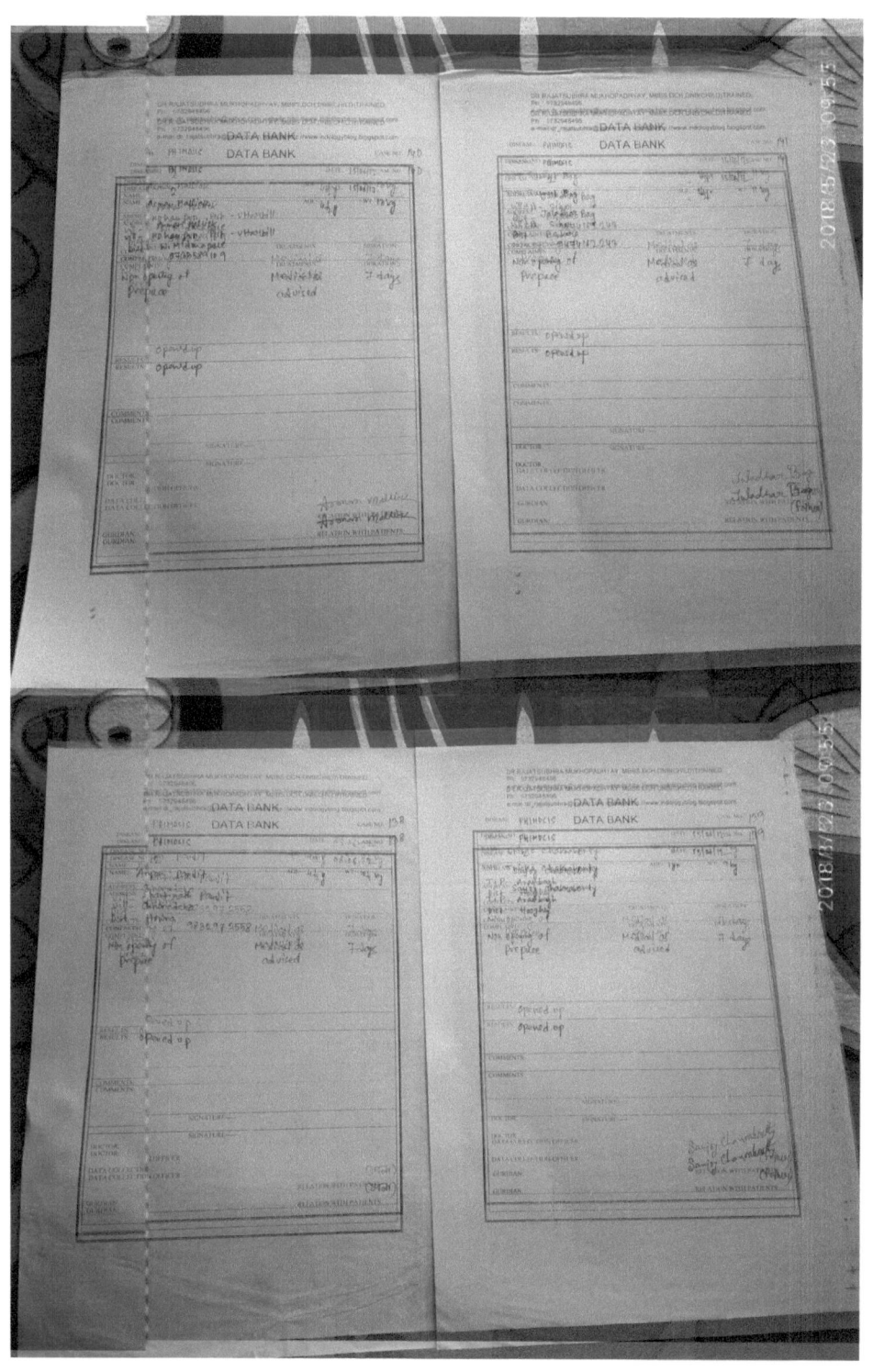

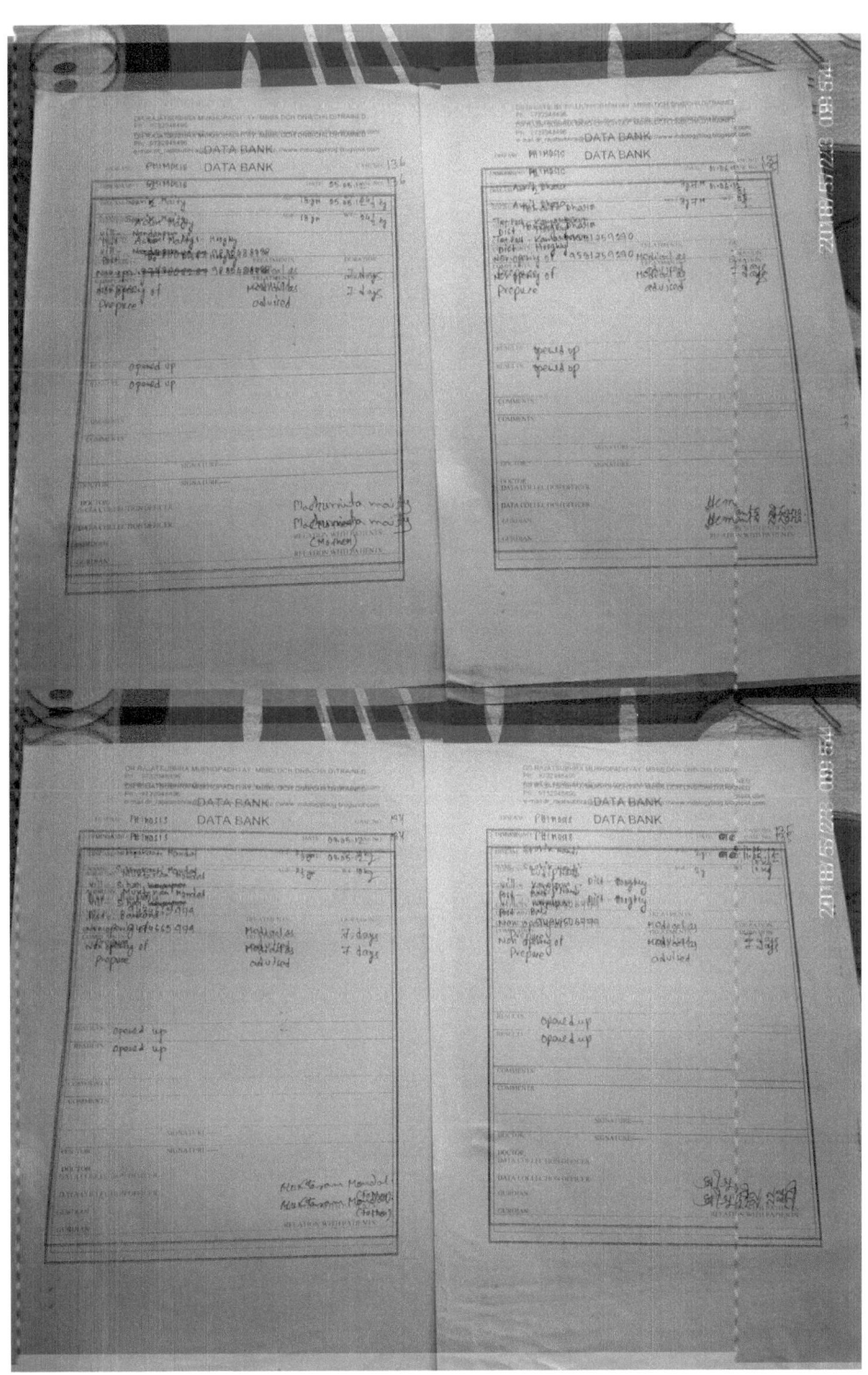

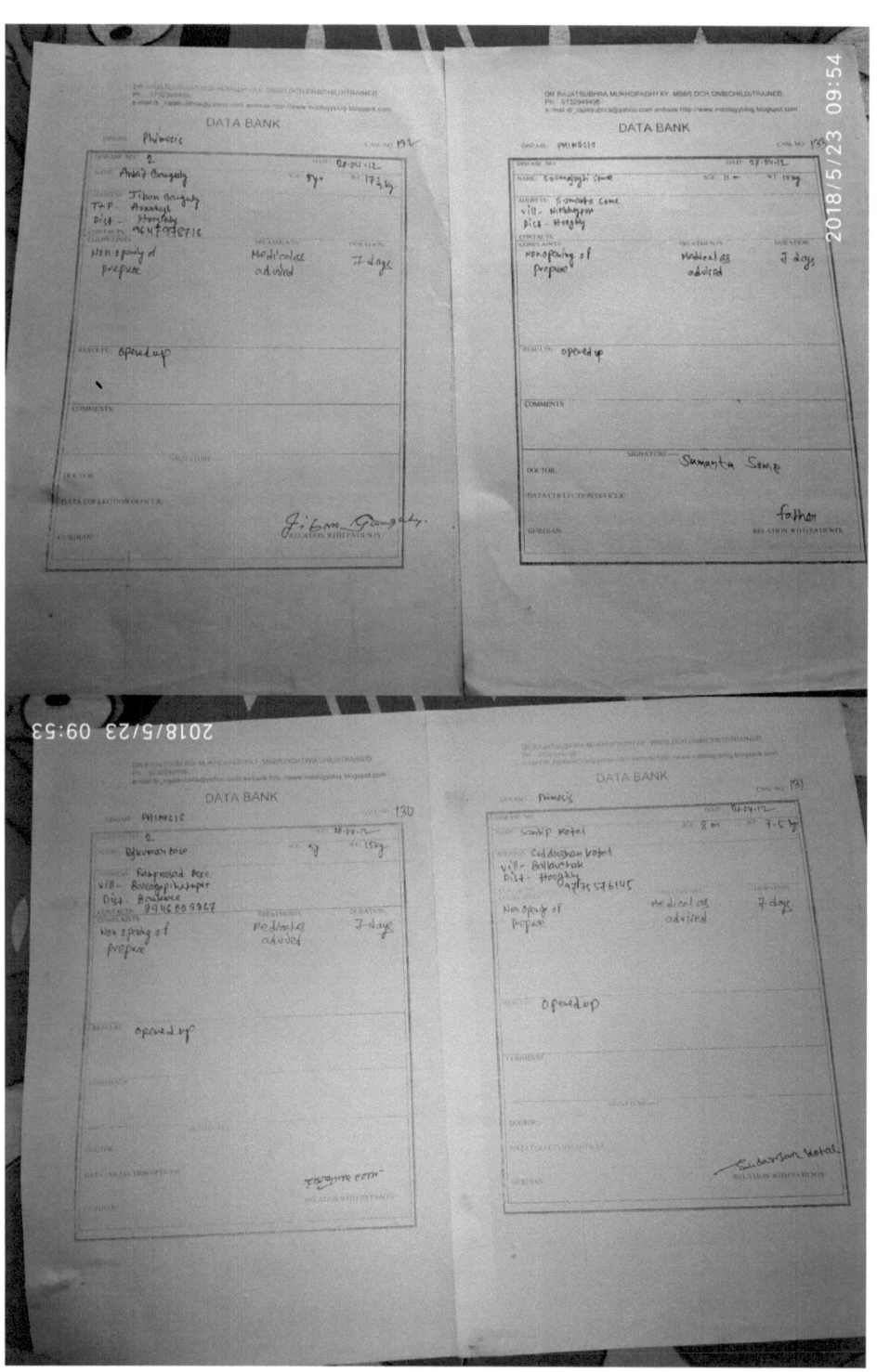

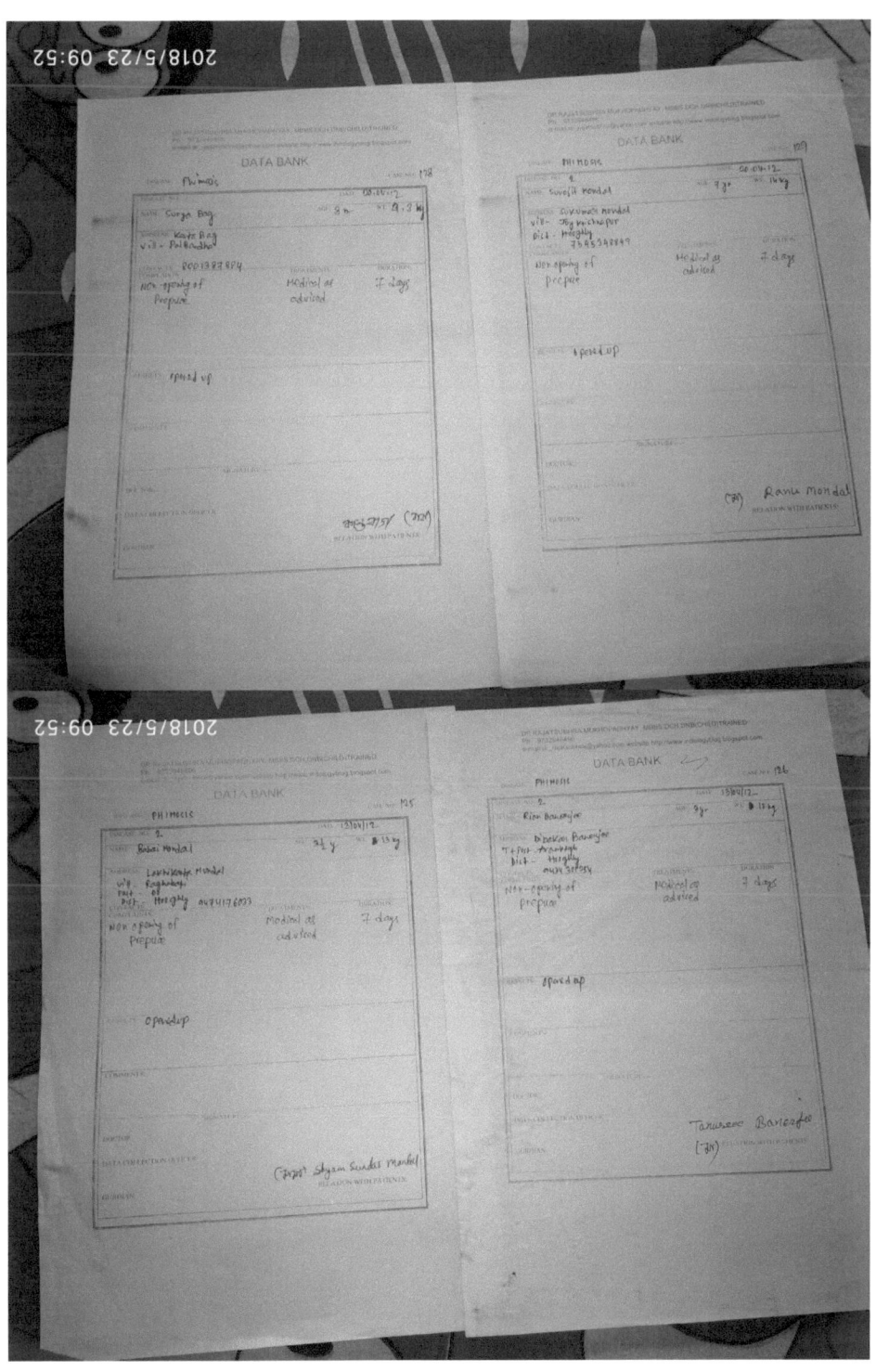

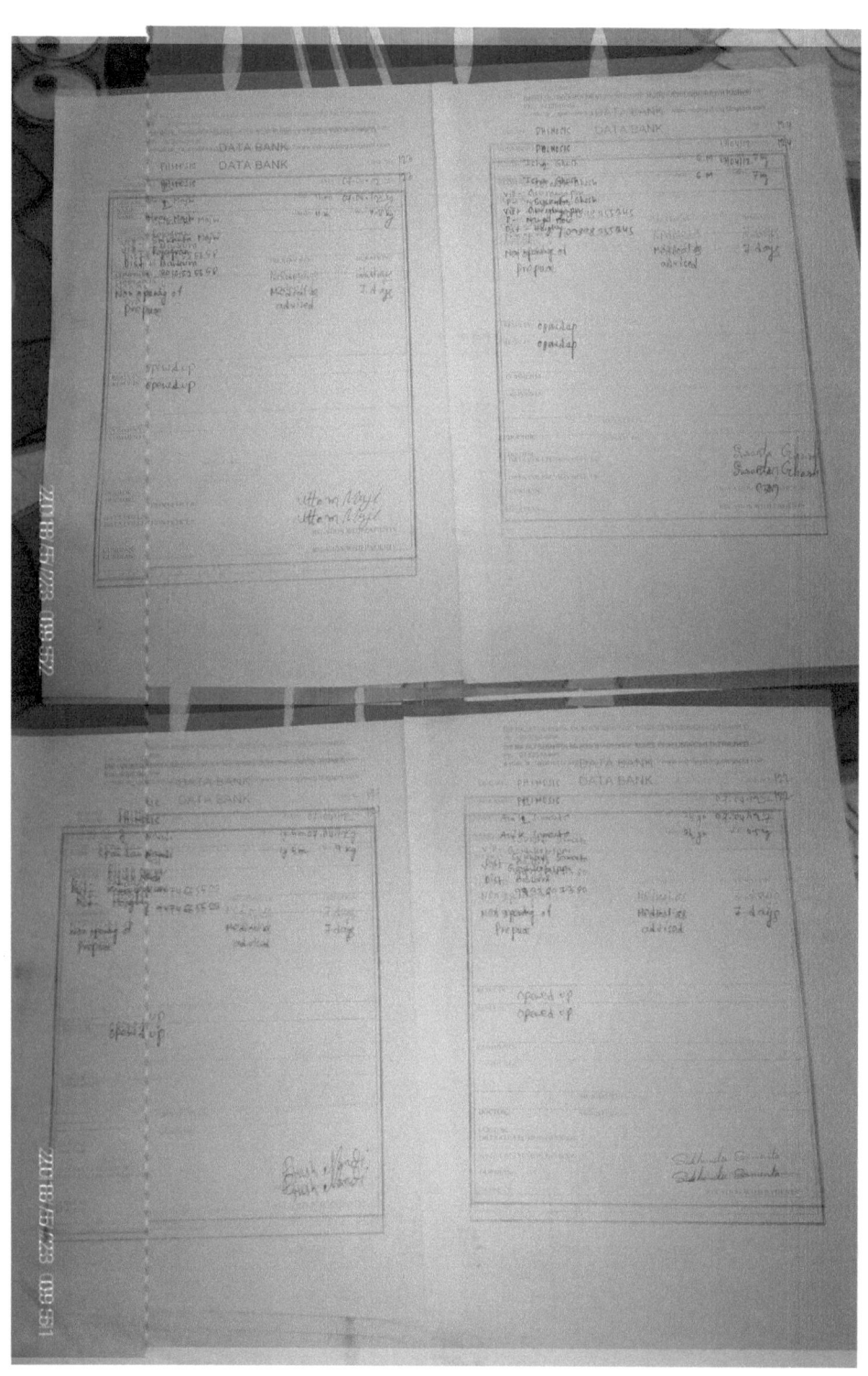

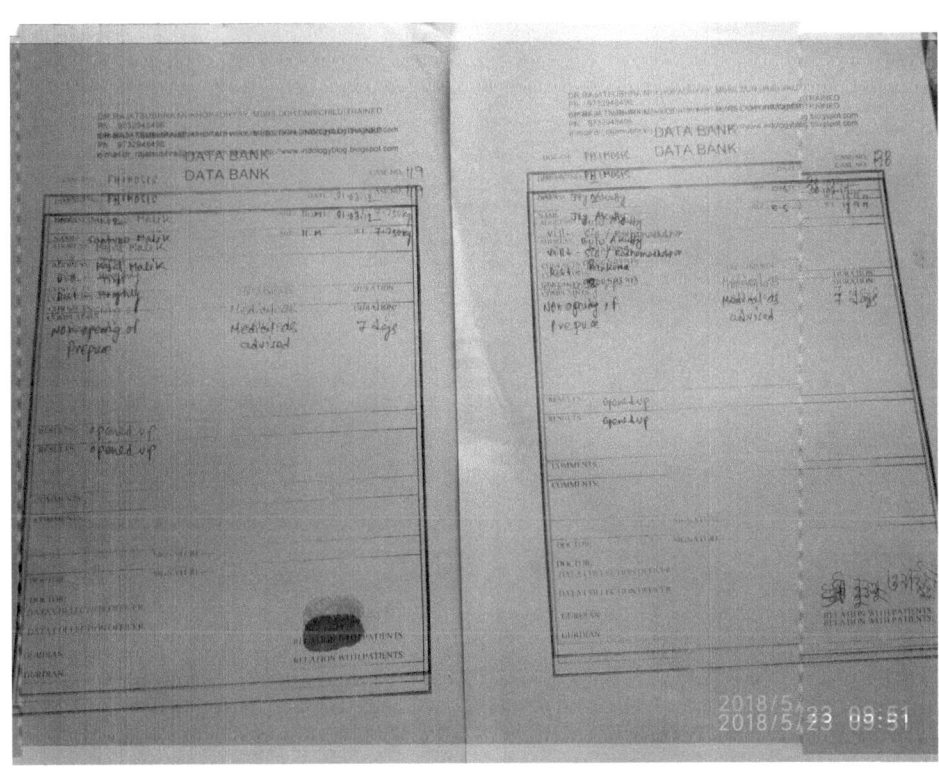

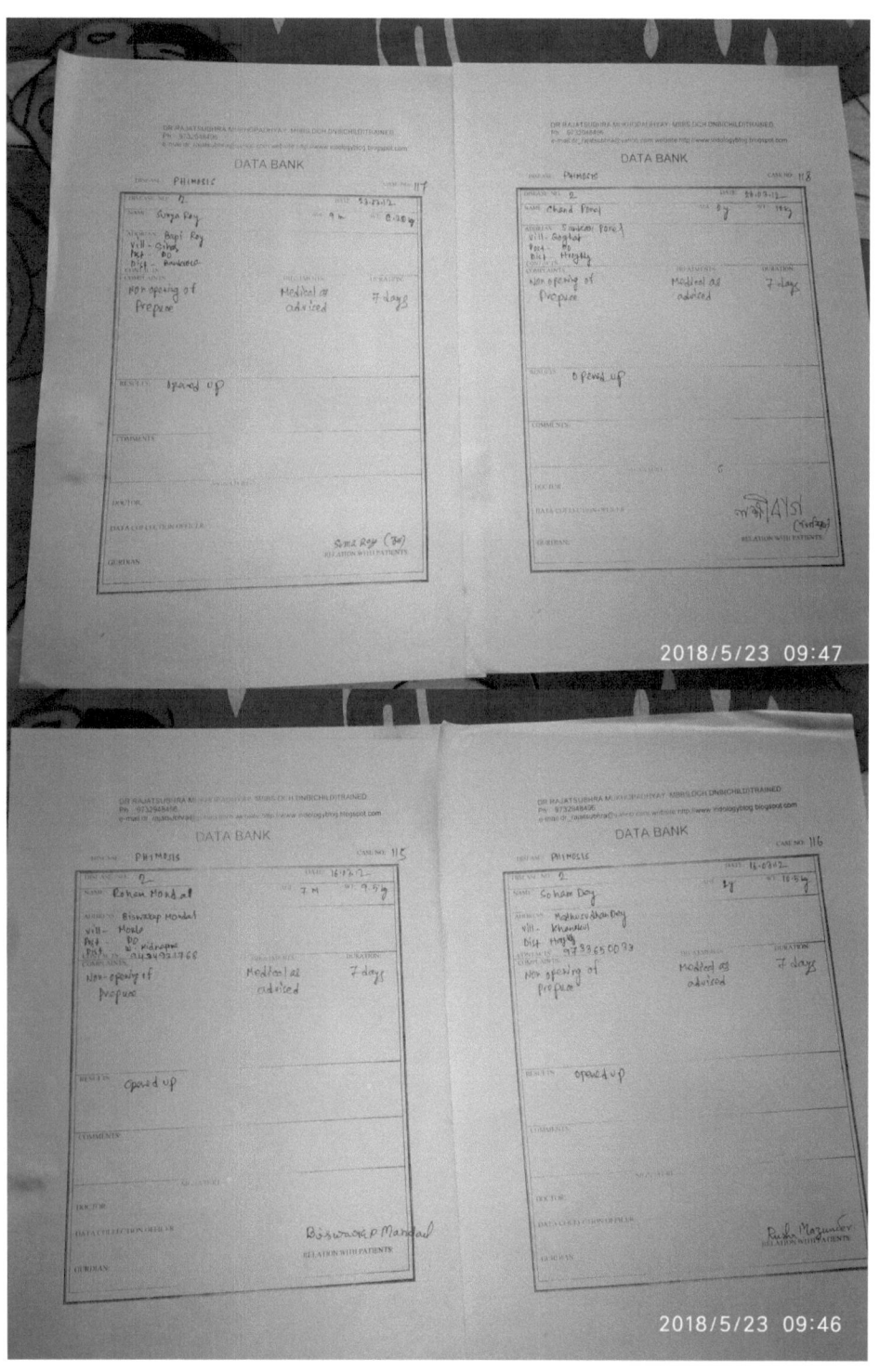

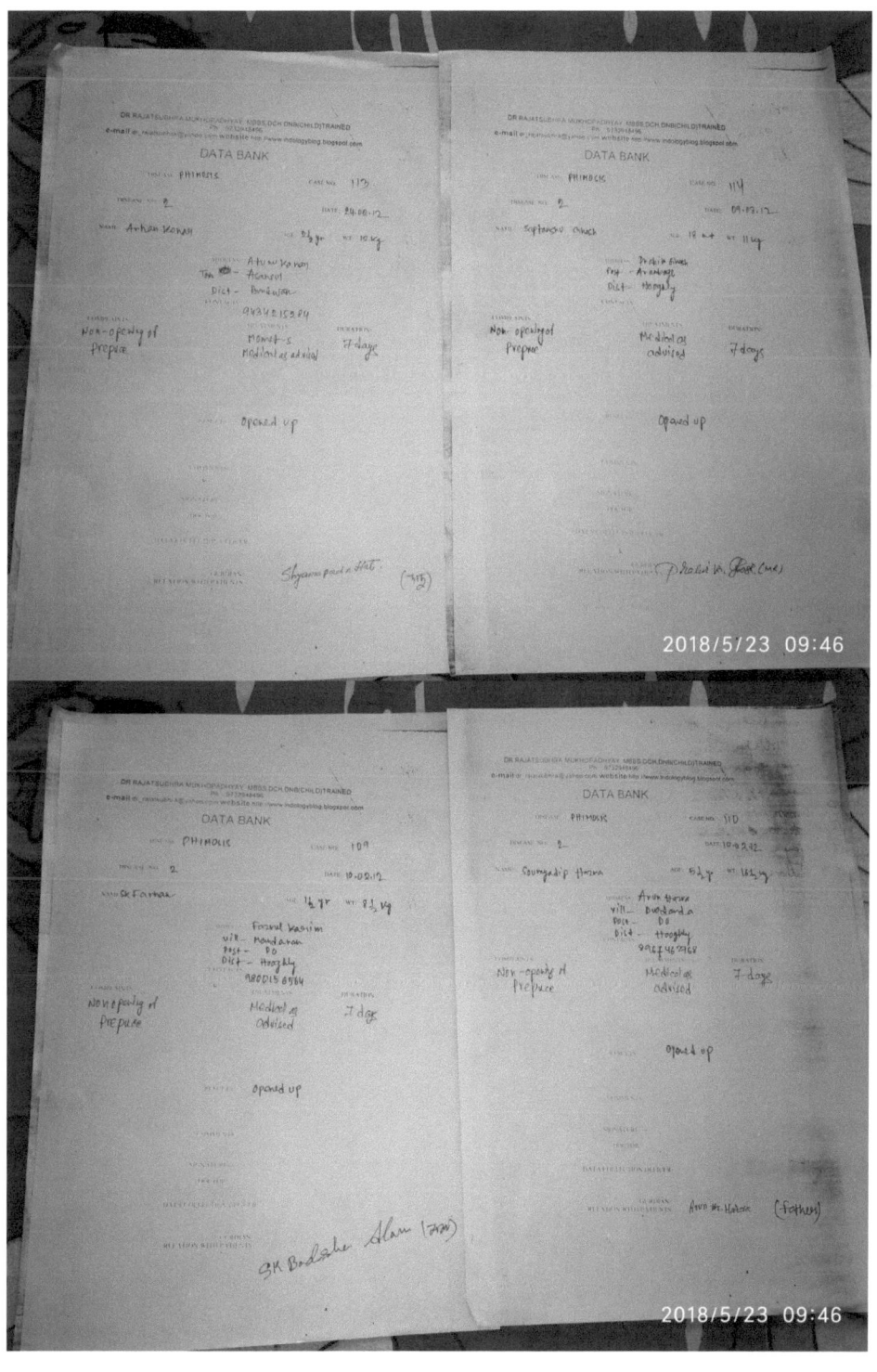

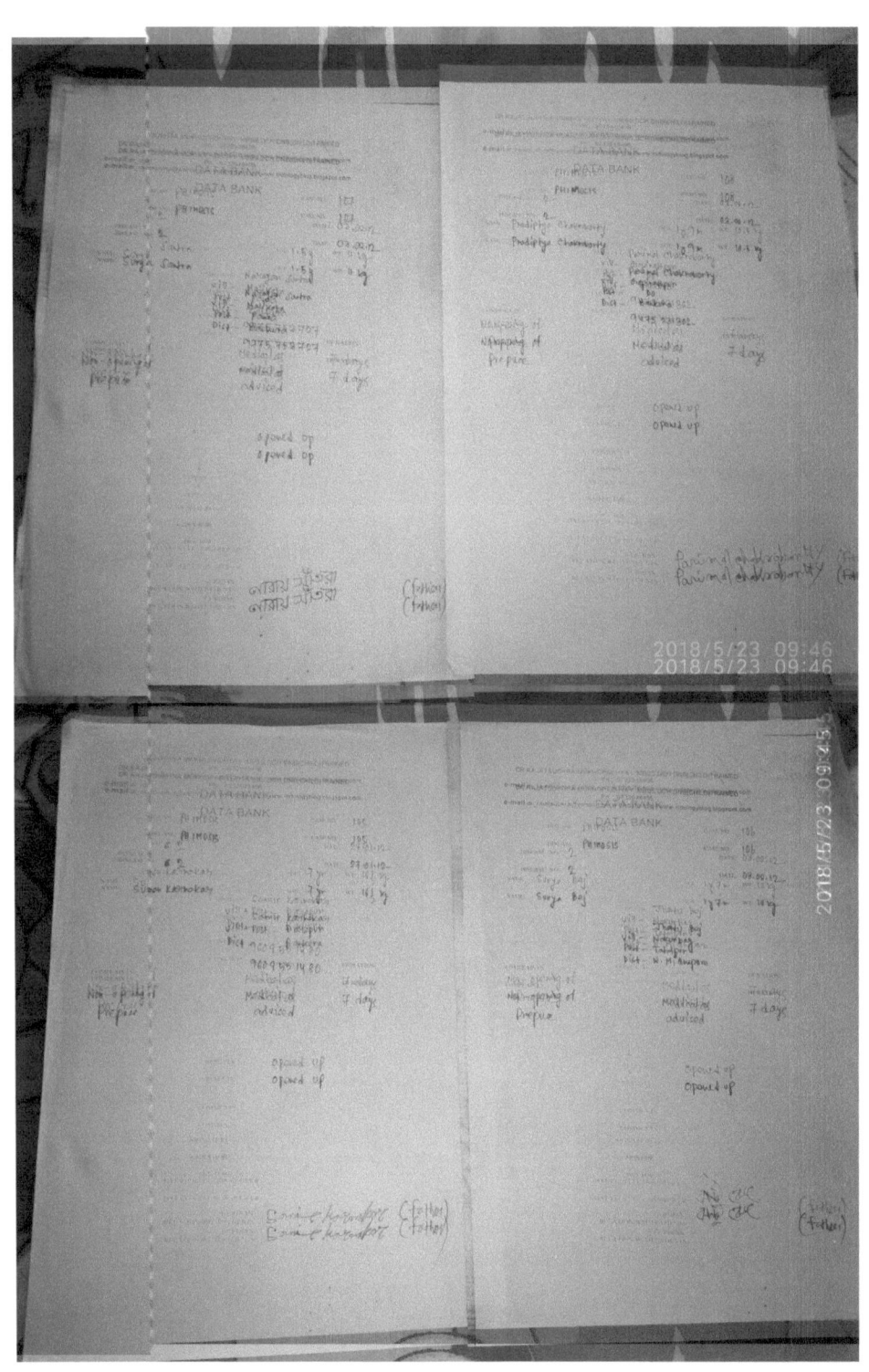

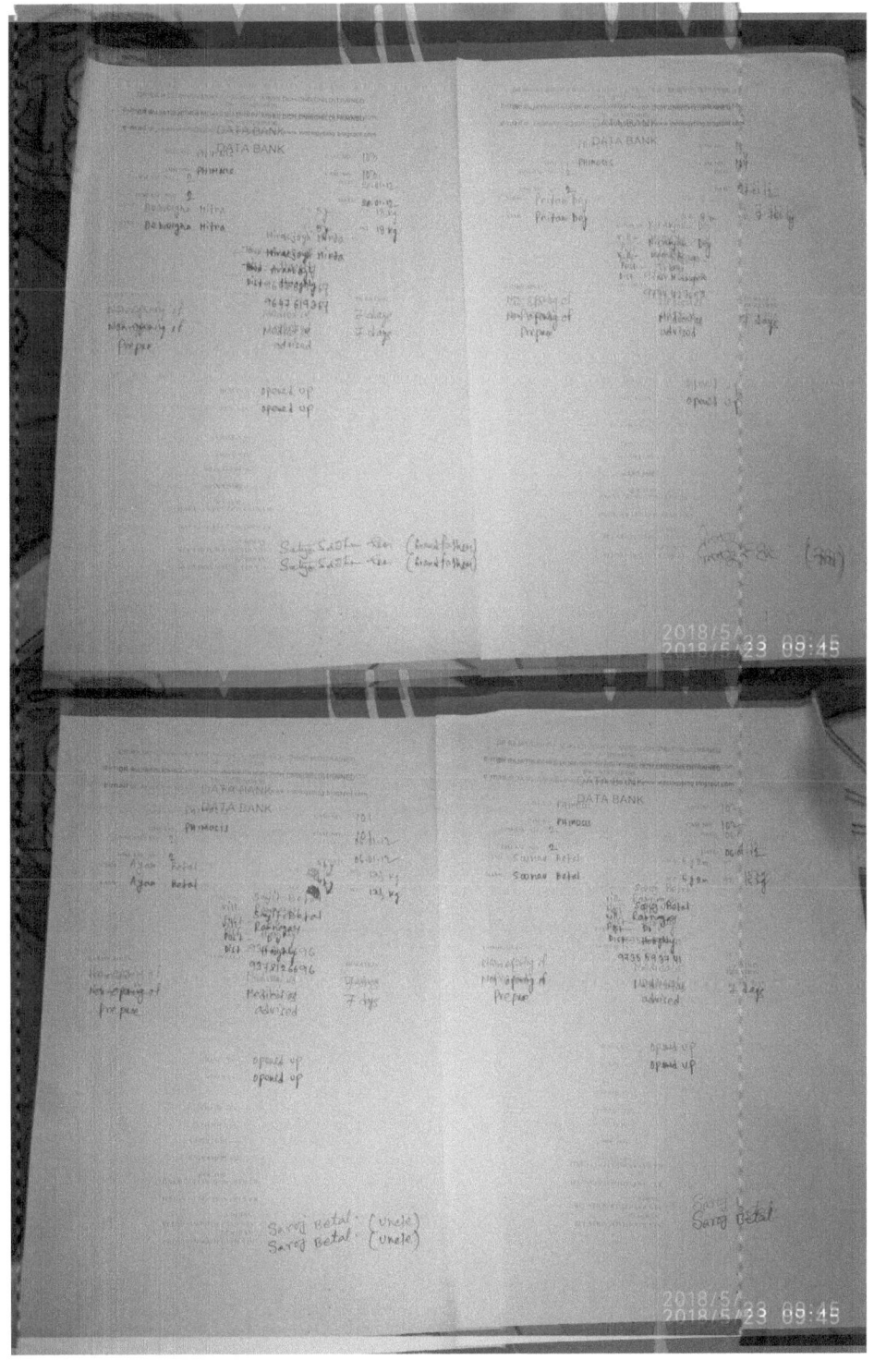

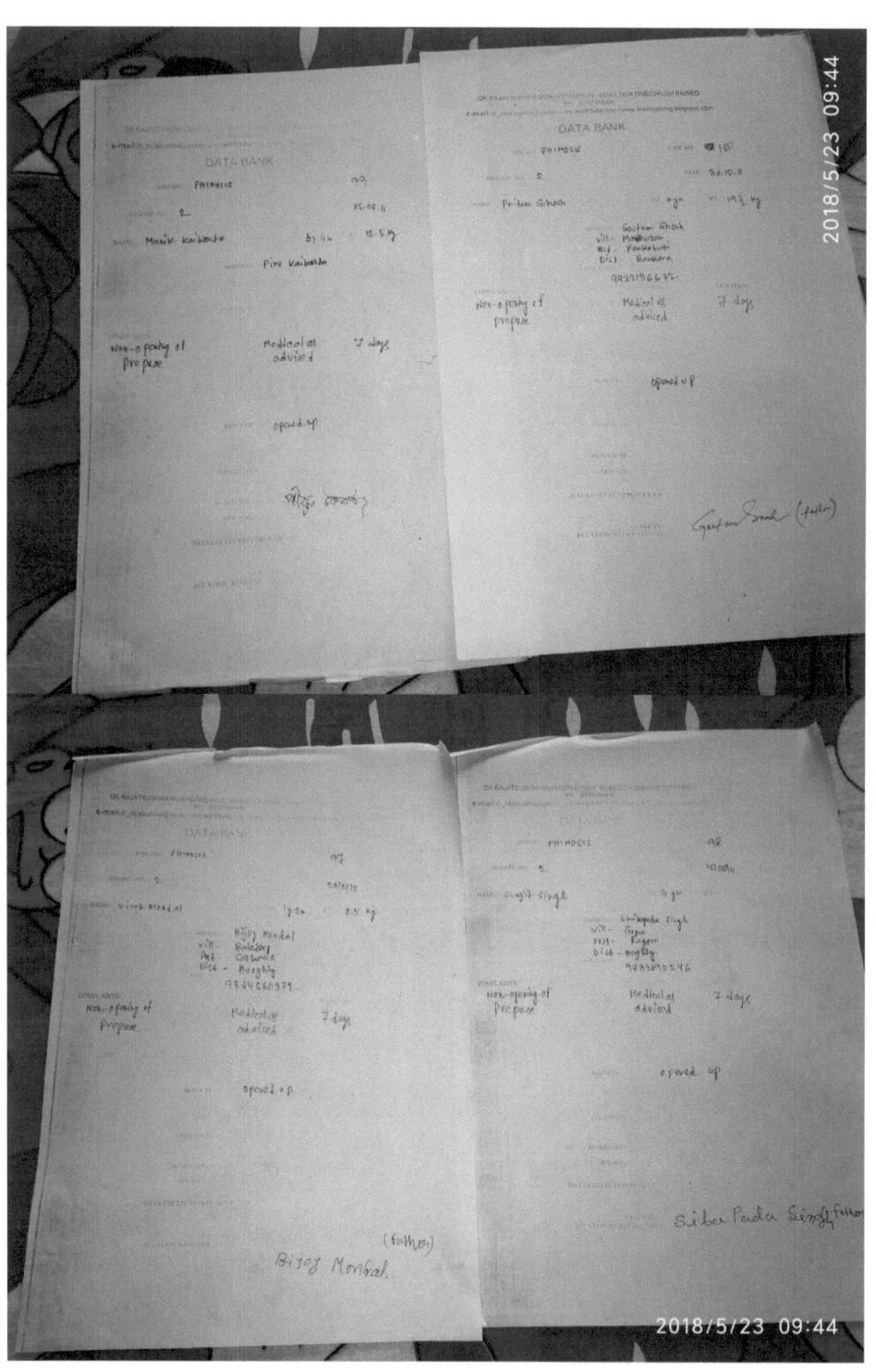

57

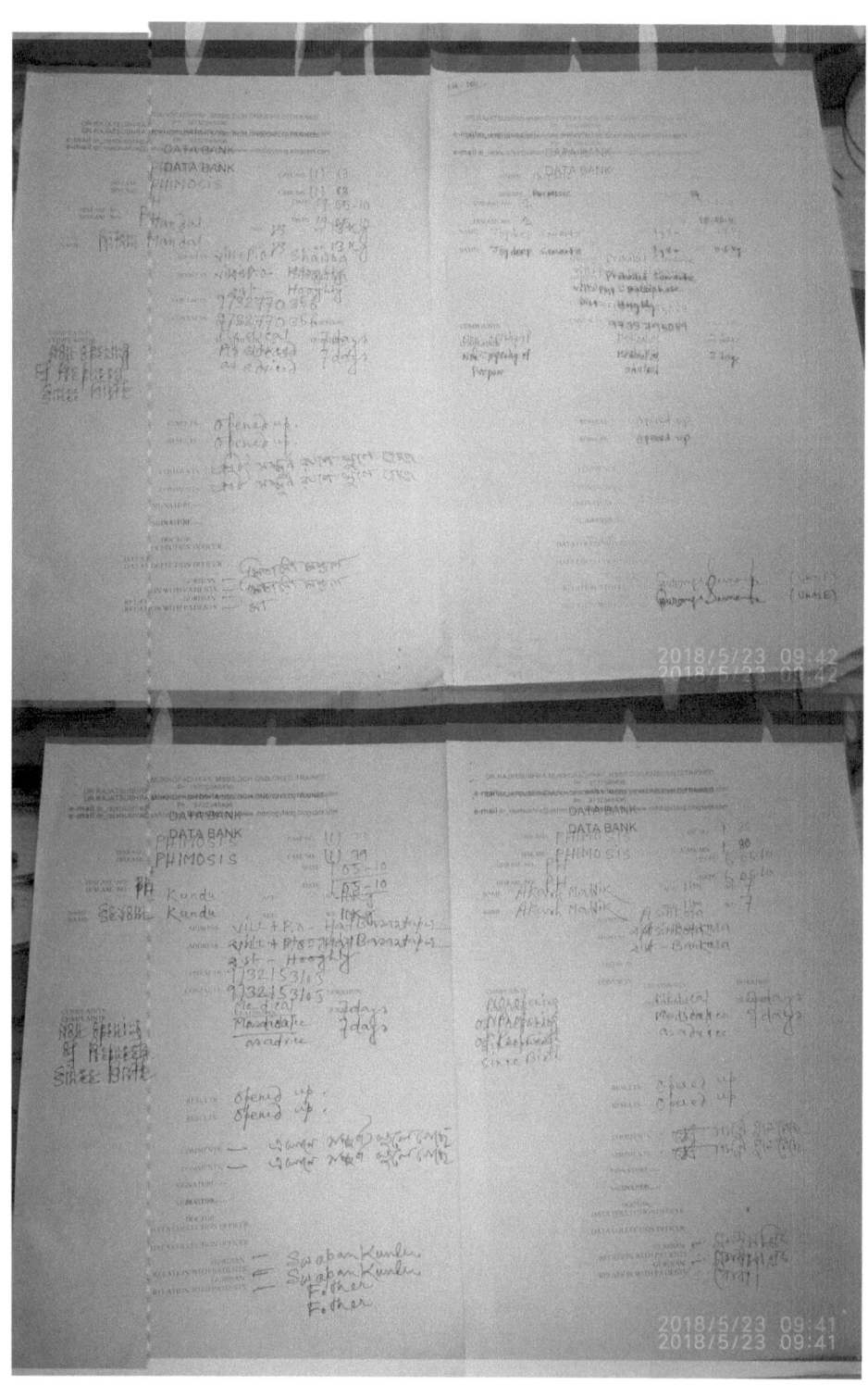

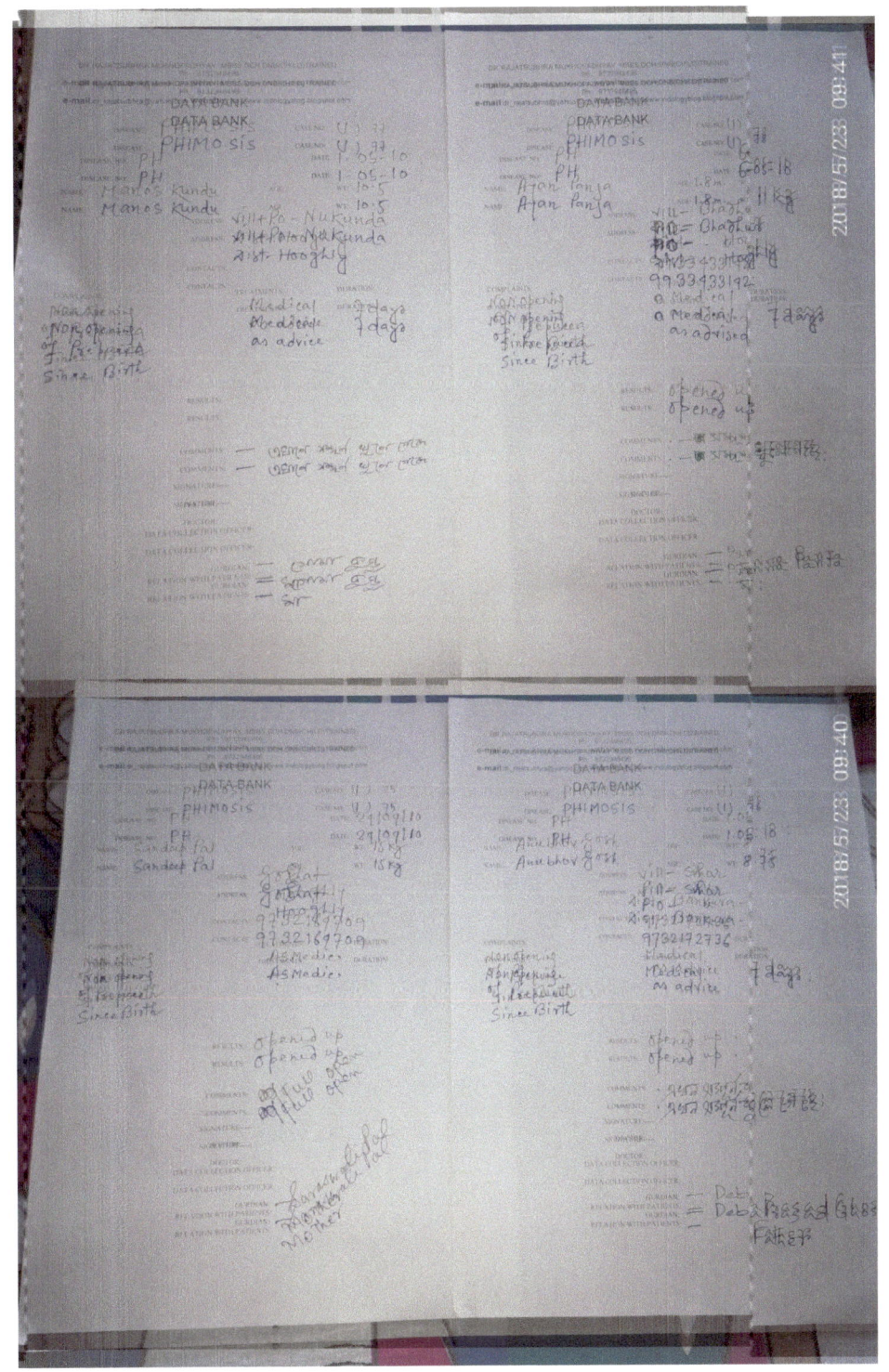

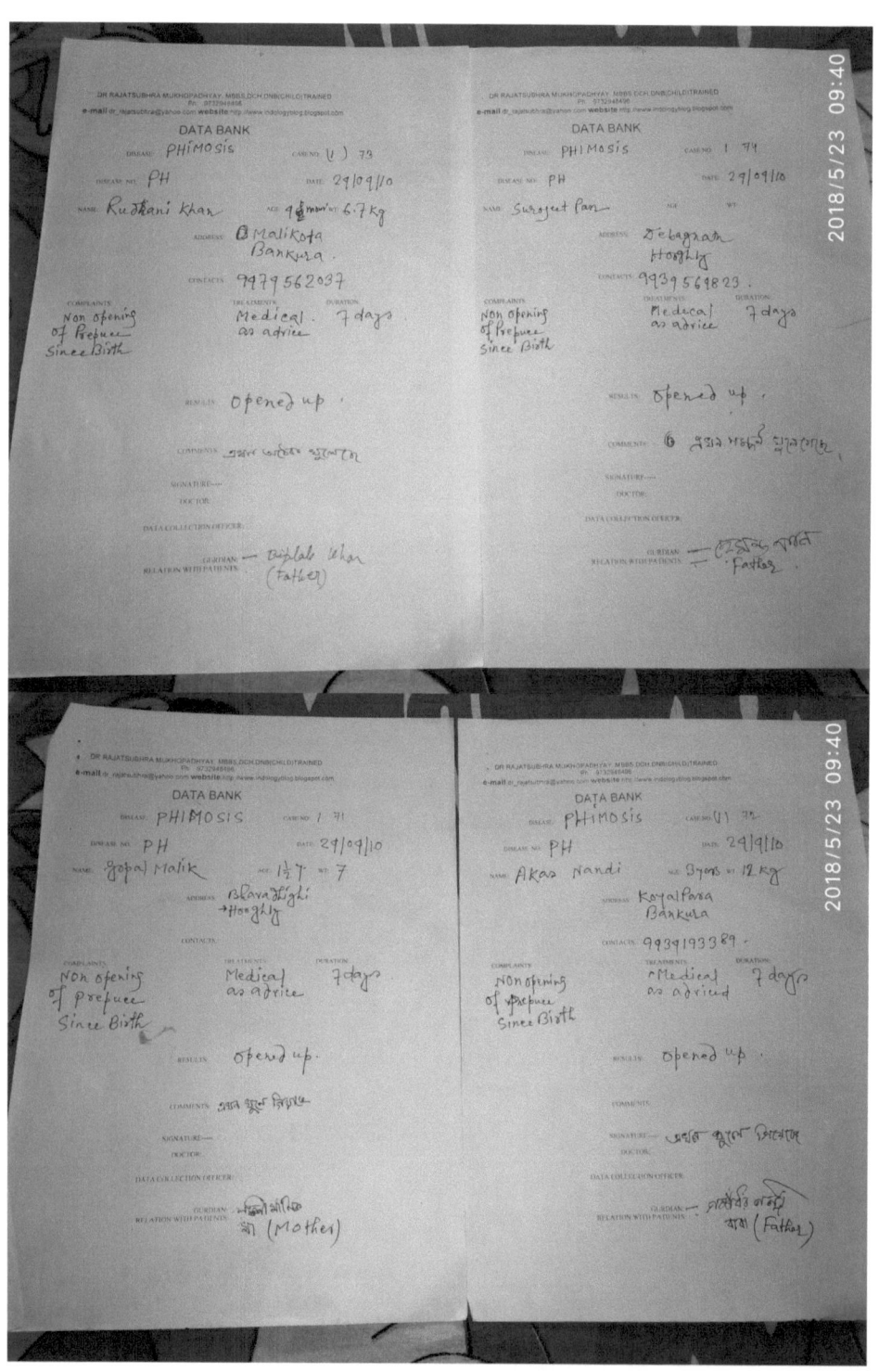

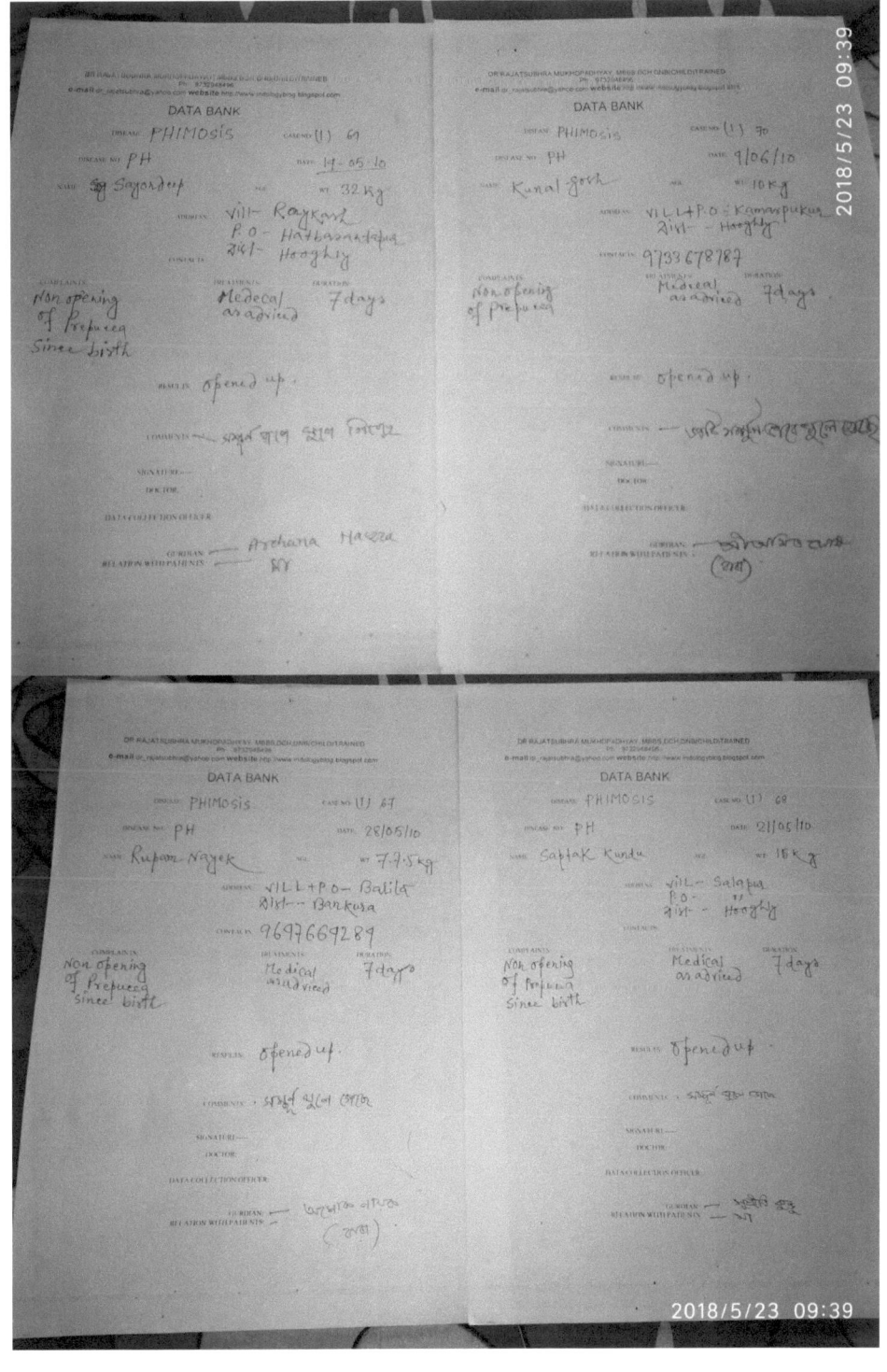

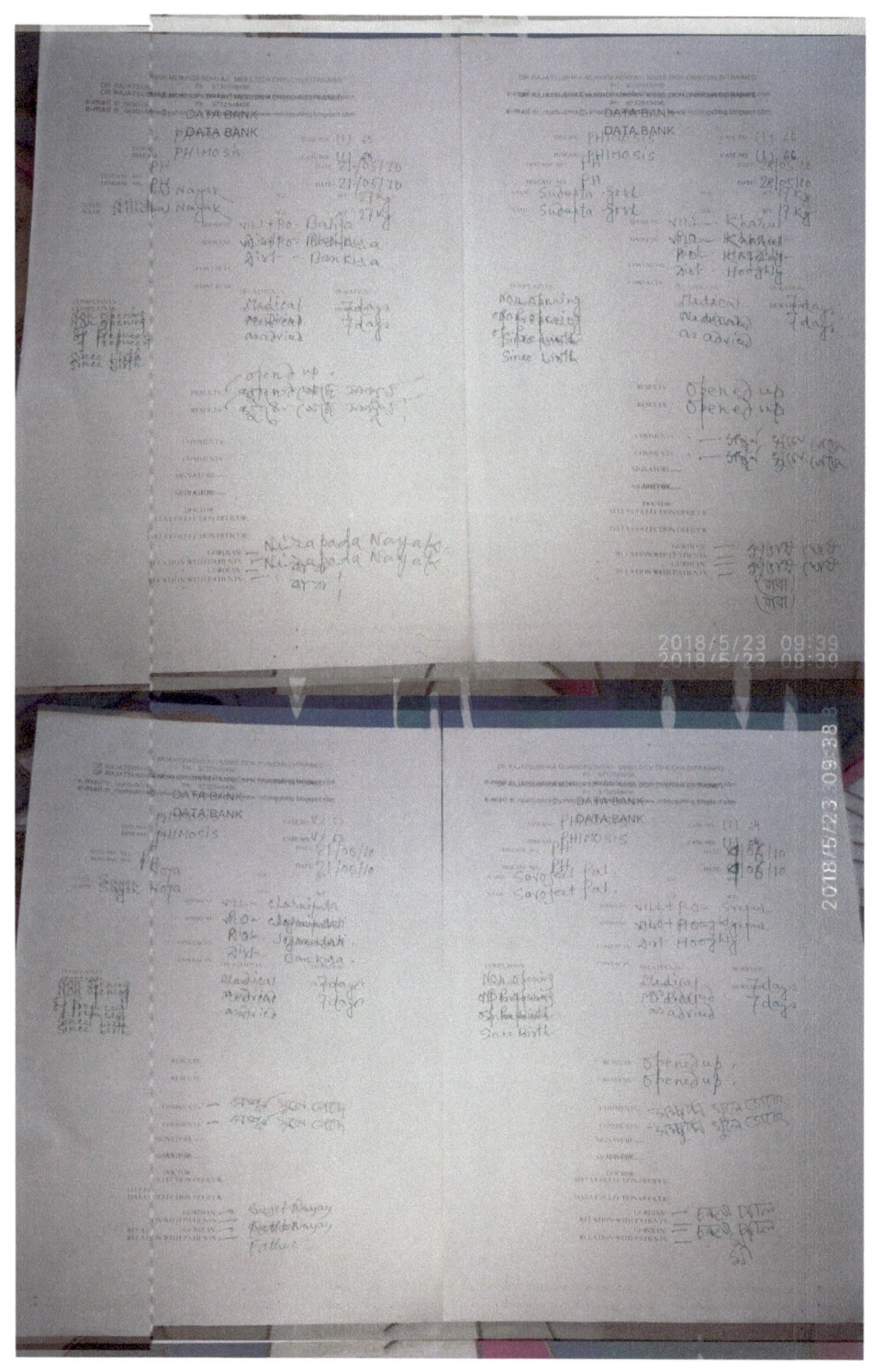

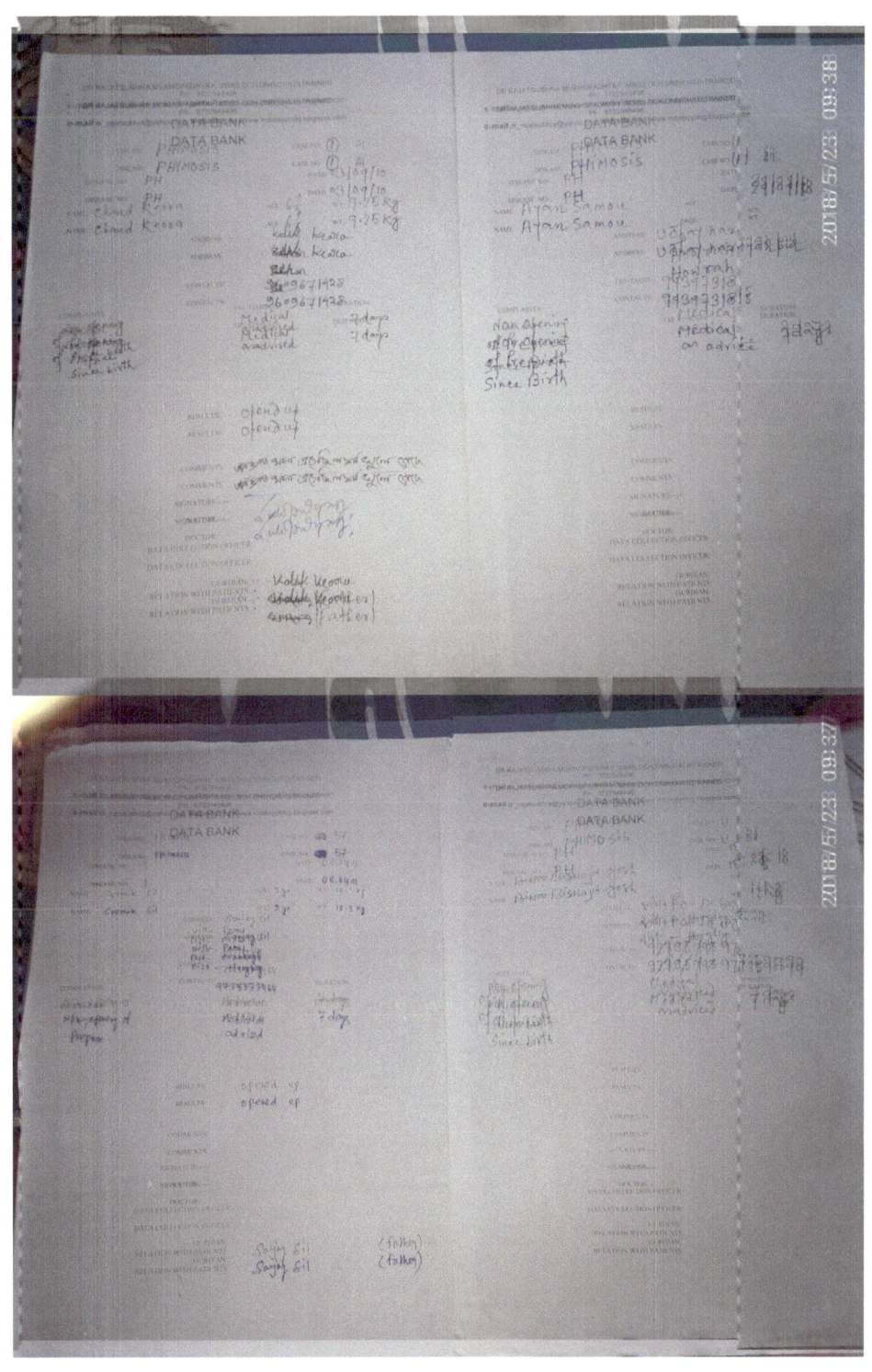

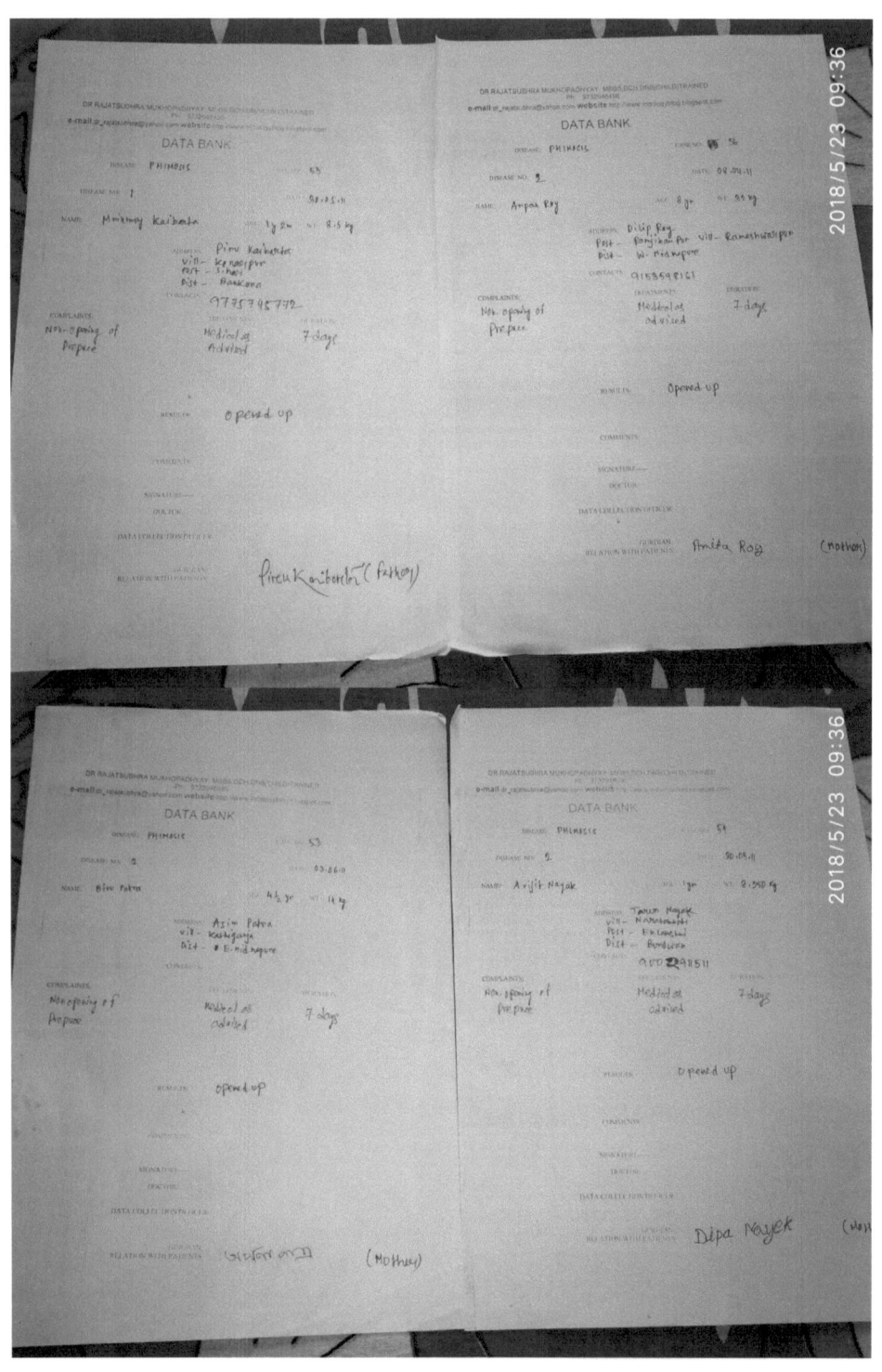

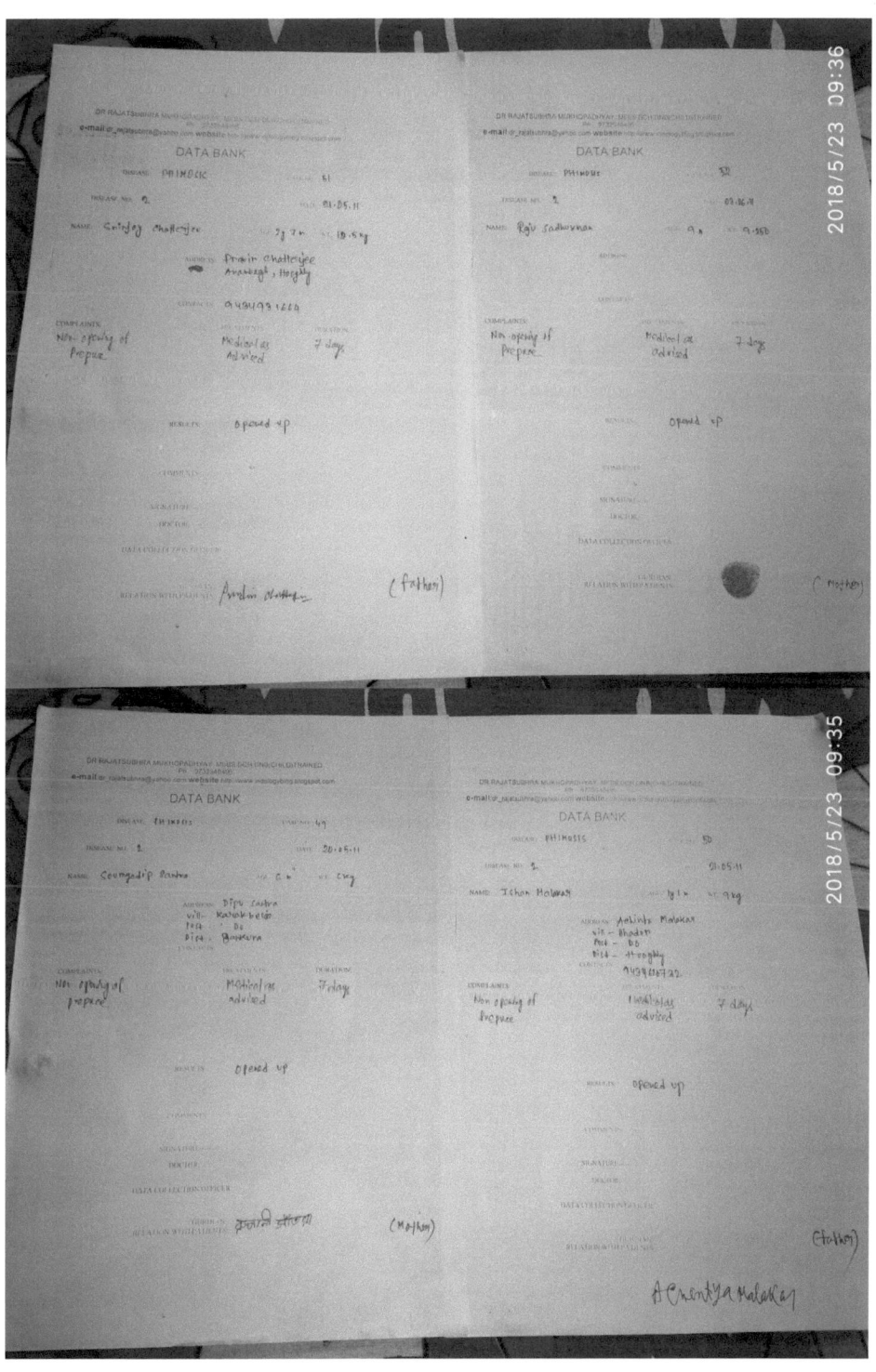

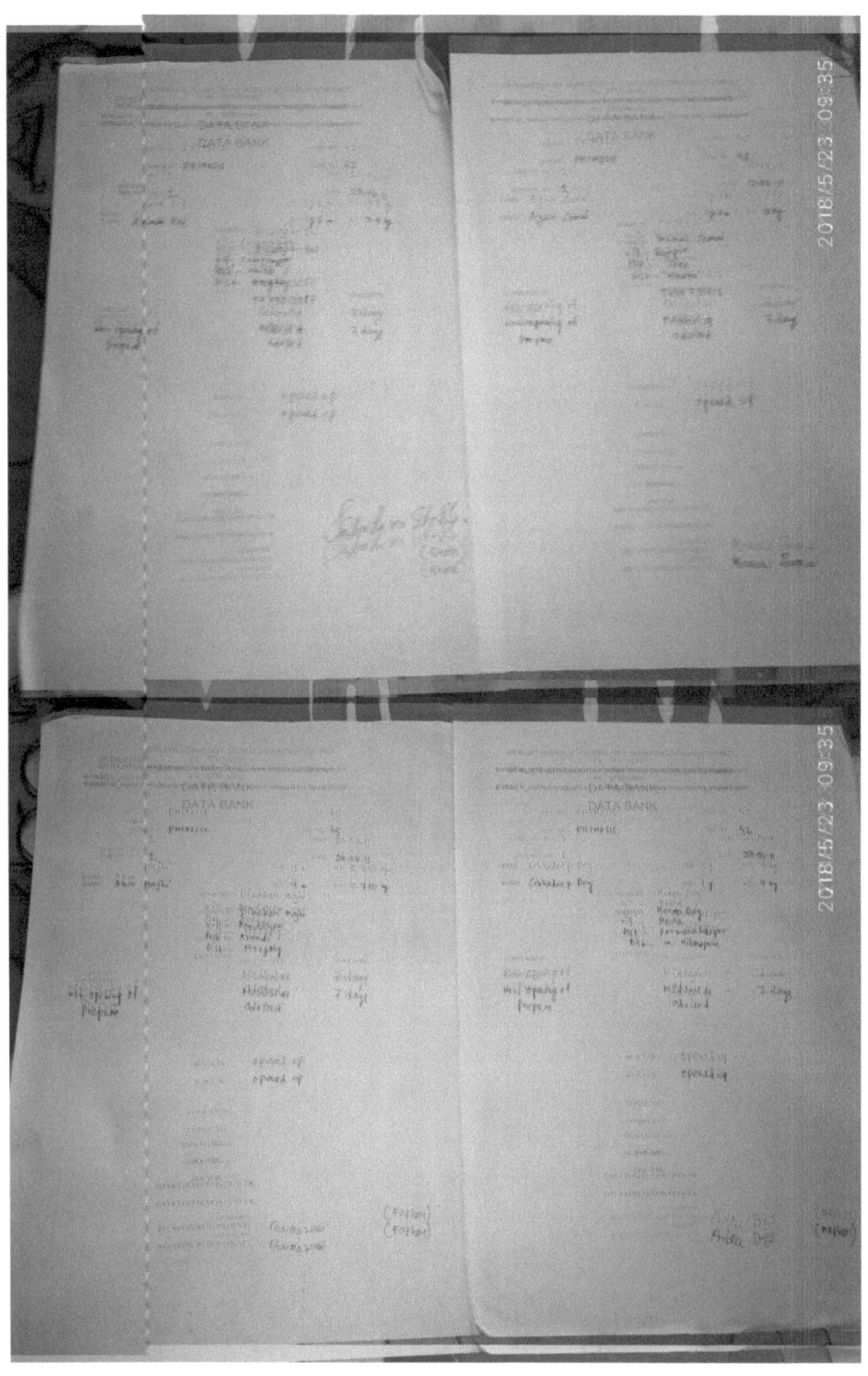

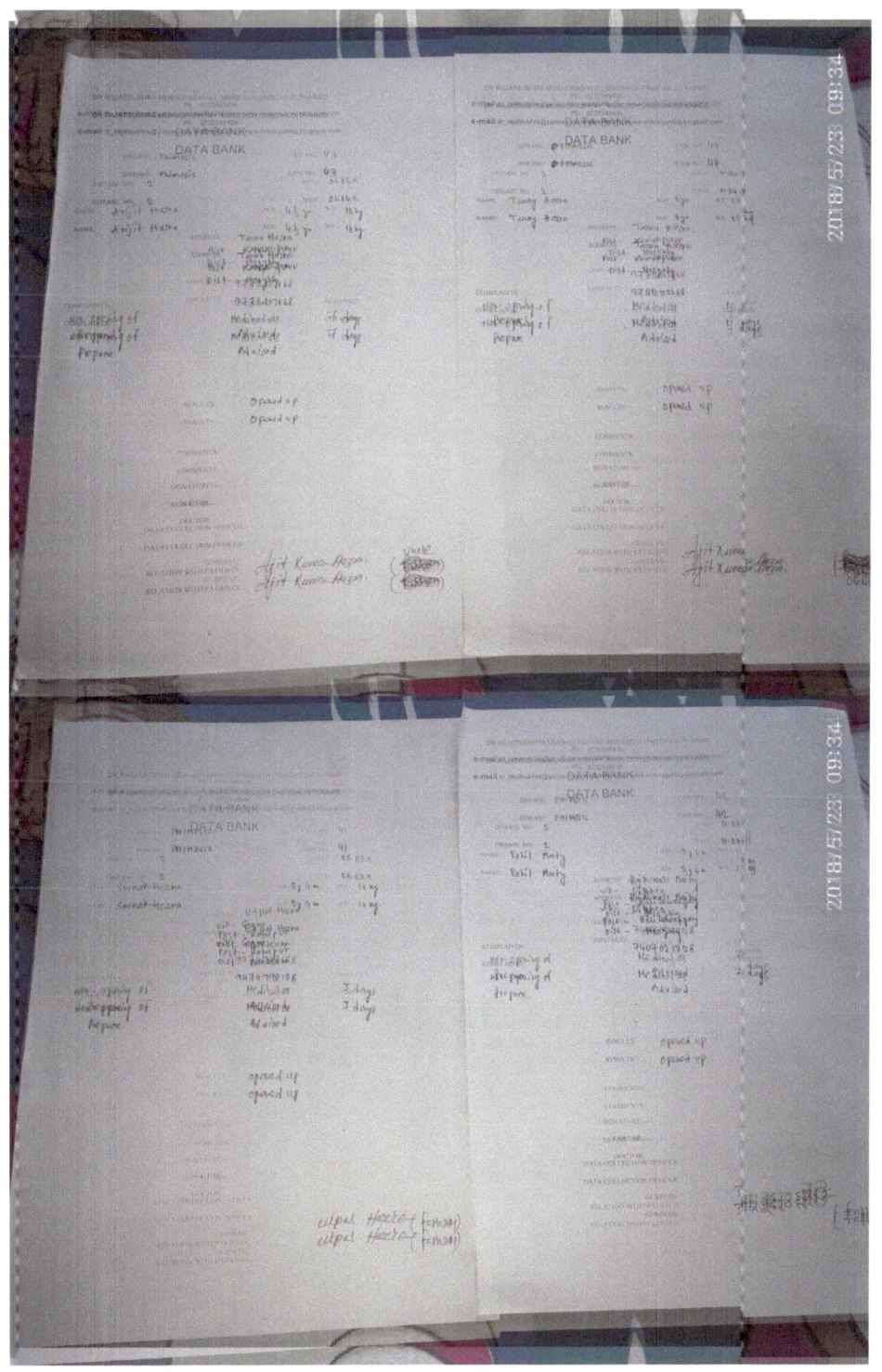

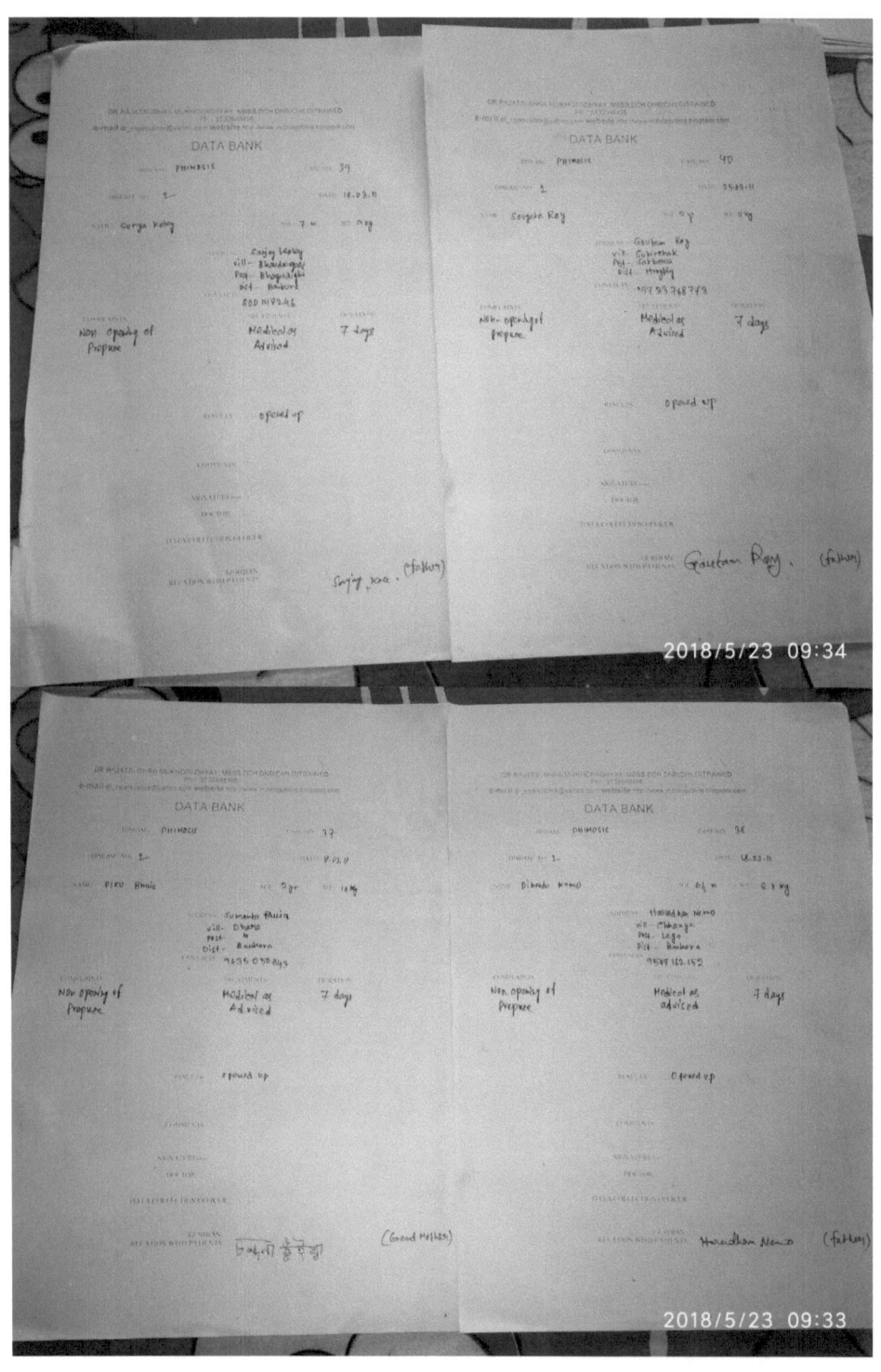

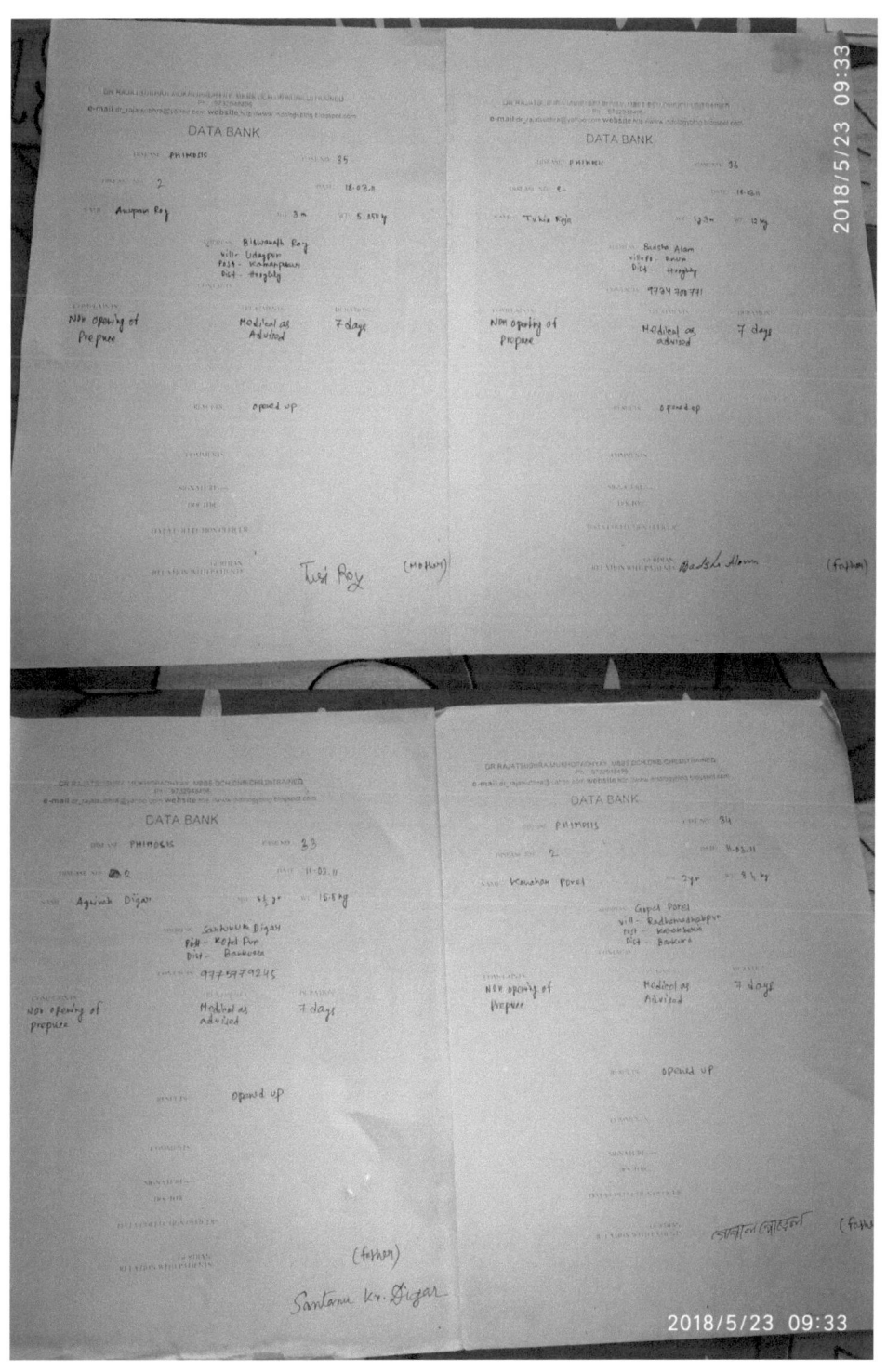

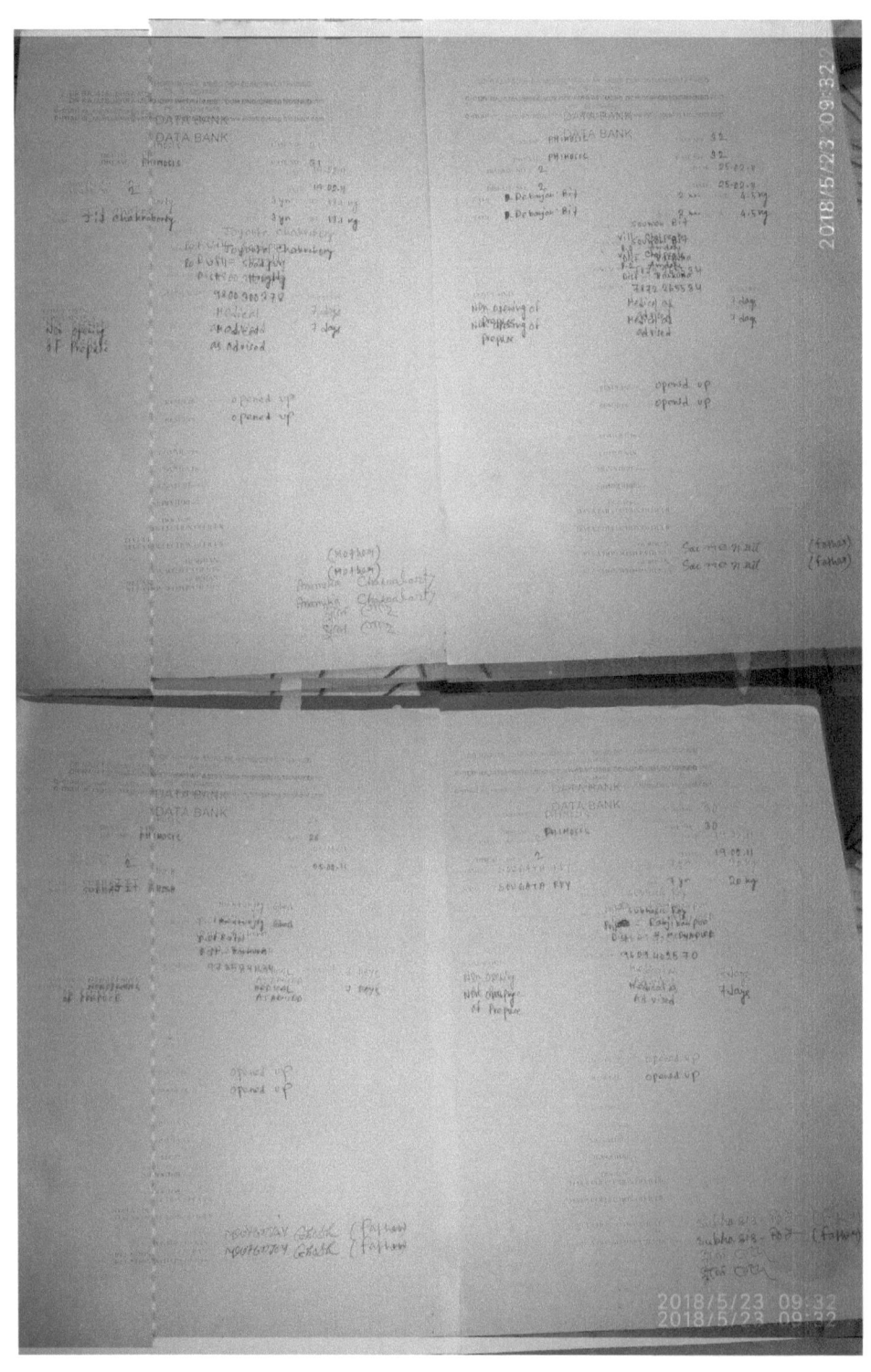

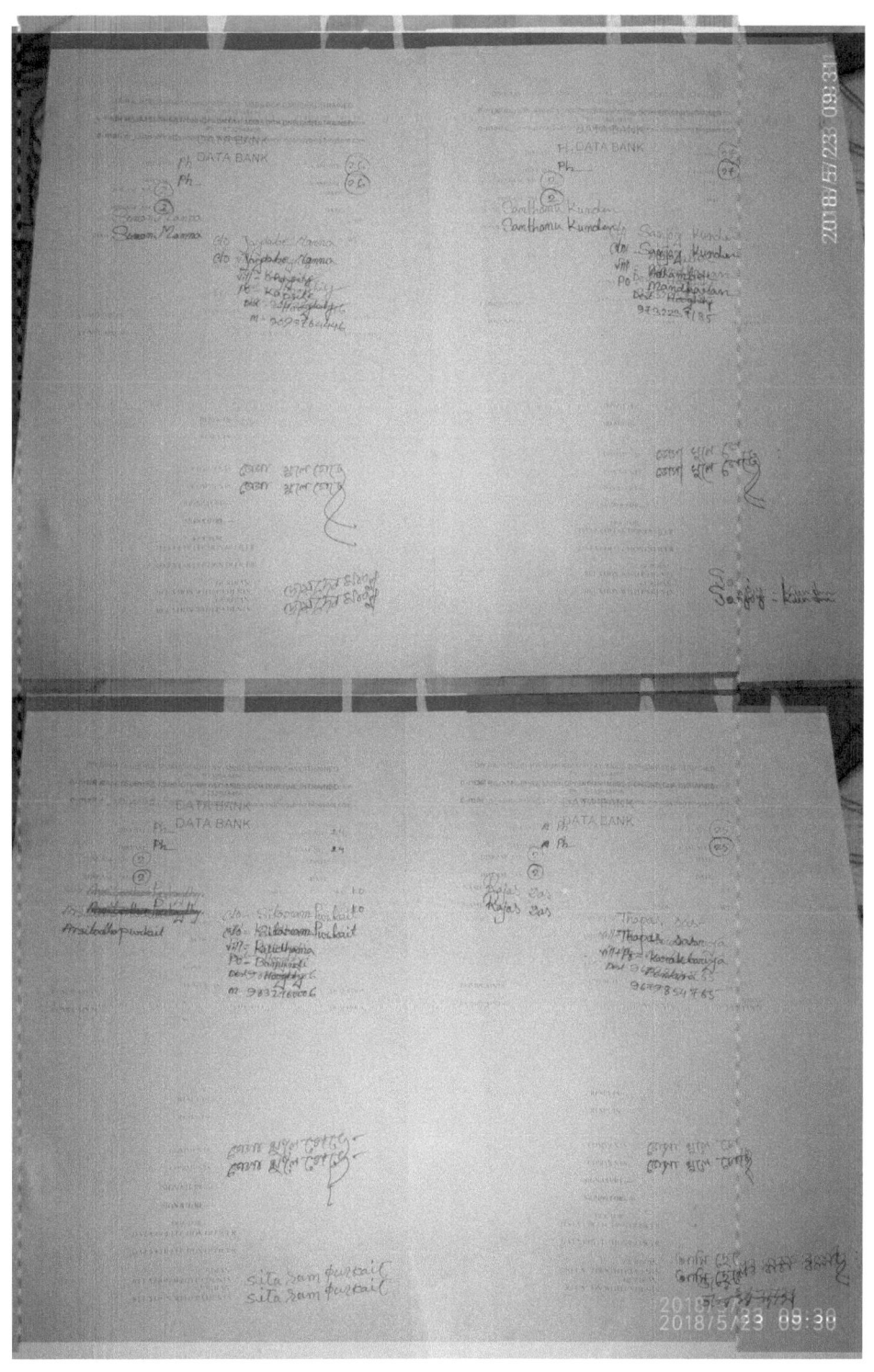

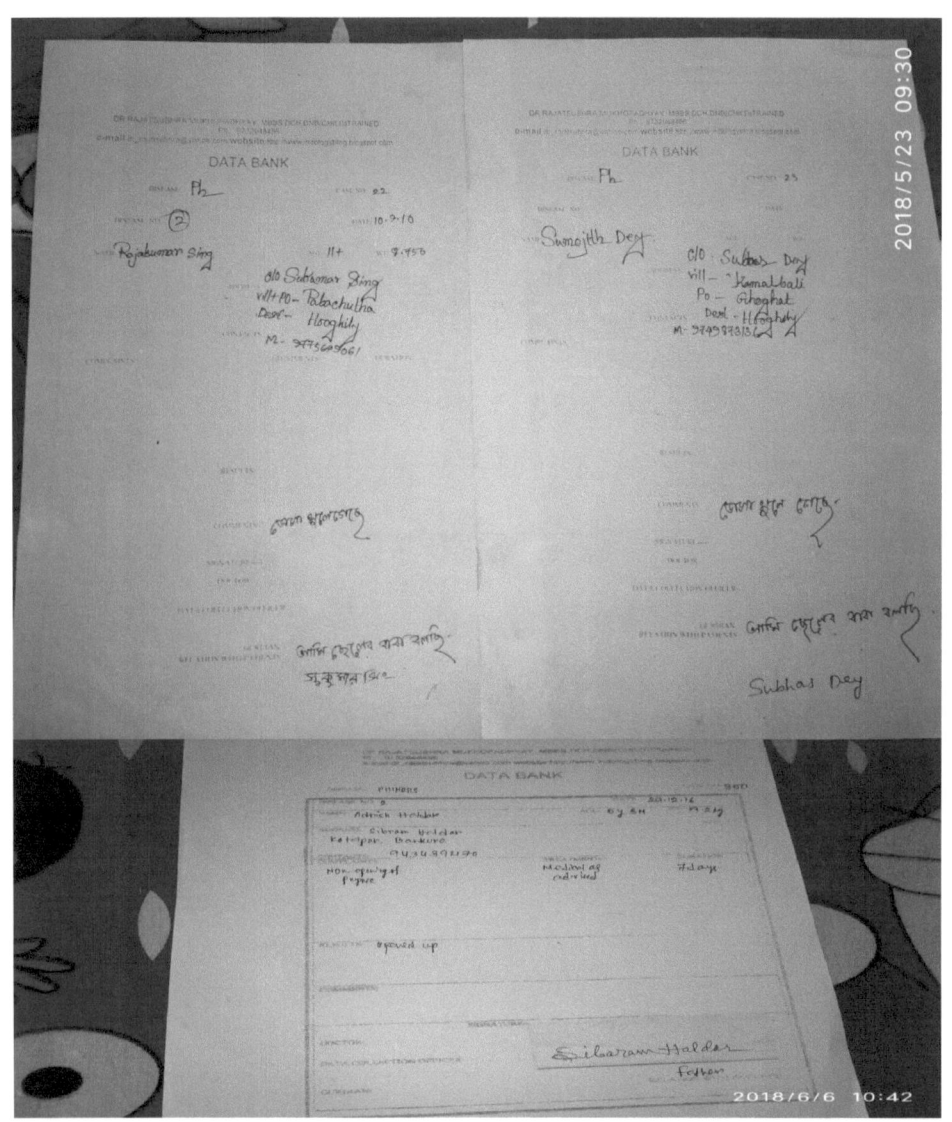

# Thank you.

From this remote rural area I need your help to continue academy and research.

I am grateful and thank you once again to all the team members of KINDLE and AMAZON.COM for proving this scope to publish my work.

Dr Rajatsubhra.

Please follow and inspire the CREATIVITY by advising to follow:
**my other books** by Amazon. https://www.amazon.in/Dr-Rajatsubhra-Mukhopadhyay-MD/e/B007HJ0F70.
My Videos in YOU Tube:
https://www.youtube.com/results?search_query=therajatsubhra
My WEB SITE: http://www.sridoctor.com
My BLOG: https://indologyblog.blogspot.com/
My Professional page in Face book:
https://www.facebook.com/Child-Health-Care-Arambag-115522941862665/

www.ingramcontent.com/pod-product-compliance
Lightning Source LLC
Chambersburg PA
CBHW051917210526
45473CB00006B/2041